Critical Reflections on Health Services Development in India

Critical Reflections on Health Services Development in India

The Teleology of Disorder

Kesavan Rajasekharan Nayar

LEXINGTON BOOKS
Lanham • Boulder • New York • Toronto • Plymouth, UK

Published by Lexington Books
A wholly owned subsidiary of Rowman & Littlefield
4501 Forbes Boulevard, Suite 200, Lanham, Maryland 20706
www.rowman.com

10 Thornbury Road, Plymouth PL6 7PP, United Kingdom

British Library Cataloguing in Publication Information Available

Library of Congress Cataloging-in-Publication Data

Nayar, K. R., 1955- author.
Critical reflections on health services development in India : the teleology of disorder / by Kesavan Rajasekharan Nayar.
p. cm.
Includes bibliographical references and index.
ISBN 978-0-7391-9206-1 (cloth : alk. paper) — ISBN 978-0-7391-9207-8 (electronic)
I. Title.
[DNLM: 1. Health Policy—trends—India. 2. Health Planning—organization & administration—India. 3. Health Services—trends—India. 4. Socioeconomic Factors—India. 5. State Medicine—organization & administration—India. WA 540 JI4]
RA418.3.I4
362.10954—dc23

2014011807

™ The paper used in this publication meets the minimum requirements of American National Standard for Information Sciences—Permanence of Paper for Printed Library Materials, ANSI/NISO Z39.48-1992.

Printed in the United States of America

Contents

Preface vii

1 Introduction: Health Services and the Domains of Disorder 1

2 Grappling with Delivery of Health Services: A Historical Examination 9

3 Reforms and Their Forms in Health Services 43

4 Centrality of Decentralization and Marginalization of the People 81

5 Civilizing the Civil Society and Civilians: Old Bottles and New Medicines 109

6 Disorder Defined: The Homogenization Process 139

References 147

Index 163

About the Author 171

Preface

This book is the product of my intensive and long-term explorations into public health which started more than three decades ago. I was trained to think like a master of all trades by my teachers who advocated that given the extreme resource constraints in developing countries, it is imperative to be well-versed with different facets of public health and diverse problems that the country is facing rather than having a narrow specialist focus fashionable in some academic disciplines in universities. I know very well that this view has pros and cons. The possible fallout of such an approach could be lack of in-depth treatment of topics when you deal with a number of issues. But I believe that this can be overcome when you are naturally inclined to approach a problem with a multi-dimensional lens and by deliberate incursions and constant churning.

Writing on a theme such as health services development of a country is most difficult especially when it has a number of dimensions and complexities and one is bound to ignore or sideline a theme which may be important to some but may be marginal to the author. This is the reason why I have deliberately chosen some essential broad factors underlining the health services with many layers and substratum that can be construed as engines for its development. The development is especially difficult to discern in a country like India where diversities across regions and states make it difficult to advance a pan Indian framework, strategy, or theory. The book is written in a style so that the whole of it or some chapters could be used as a reading for public health courses as well as a resource book for generating further insights and research in the area of health services development.

Knitting together such layers or substratum is challenging and requires perseverance sometimes difficult to achieve in a work culture which does not support creative endeavors wholeheartedly. Despite all odds, I could take this to a logical end with some degree of satisfaction. I am indeed grateful to a number of individuals for this. Foremost are my family—Tara, Ammu, and Ranjith who provided all the support and a source of strength. I am also greatly indebted to my students who stood with me and helped me by providing research assistance, technical, and moral support. This book is dedicated to all of them.

Kesavan Rajasekharan Nayar

1

Introduction

Health Services and the Domains of Disorder

The health service is a socio-technical institution shaped by a number of actors and a multitude of interests. Despite the dominance of a techno-centric approach to public health universally and nationally, there exits an alternate vision to public health which considers health services as a social and cultural institution. Health services and health service development need to be conceptualized as a system having a number of dimensions and therefore there is a need for a systems approach to study health services–people interphase (Banerji, 1986). Three components can be identified in this alternate paradigm:

> The problems of health of a community and the cultural responses to these problems are the functions of ecological conditions shaped by the modes of production and production relations.
>
> Issues of health status and health services development are basically political issues such as the pattern of socio-economic development including nutrition, sanitation, housing, etc. Allocation of resources and choice of technology are also political issues. Politics also determines access of communities to health care.
>
> Socio-cultural factors which set a limit to possibilities of political action and purposive interventions to improve health services form the third dimension.

Banerji argues that these three components form the essence of an alternative approach to what he calls the New Public Health (Banerji, 1986:148-150). There is a need to distinguish between health system and health service system in terms of their dimensions (Qadeer, 2011). Health system according to Qadeer "is a dynamic concept embracing biological and social dimensions of the well-being of a person. On the other hand, health services system is a complex of research, education, and delivery systems (for preventive, promotive, and rehabilitative services) and is only one of the many inputs required to improve the health of the people" (Qadeer, 2011: 63). The two systems are important for understanding social determinants and to grapple with the problem of health of the people within this framework which can be called as critical public health. However, different approaches are needed for undertaking empirical studies as both systems have distinct social-political-technological subsystems. For instance, an epidemiological and managerial approach is more important for studying the health services system while a predominantly social science and epidemiological approach is needed for the health system. The health of the people is influenced by the inter-phase between the two systems in all their complexity with epidemiology providing the connecting link (Nayar and Priya, 2007). Health service system is also influenced by a number of organizational imperatives and a number of actors also play an important role in shaping it. Prominent among the actors within the health service system are the State represented by both bureaucratic and technocratic organizations, the civil society especially the NGOs and other organizations involved in health care, and the people who are the beneficiaries of the services. Such a complex and comprehensive definition of health and health services was perhaps missing in many earlier definitions of health system which is comprised of organizations, institutions, and resources for improving and maintaining health (Hunter, 2008). An understanding of such a system will be limited by the key functions such as stewardship (oversight and governance), financing (revenue collection, fund pooling, and purchasing), service delivery (for personal and non-personal health services), and resource generation (investment in personnel, inputs, and technologies).

As against this purely organizational vision, it is now well-accepted, given the behavioural, cultural, institutional, sociological, economic, historical, and political facets of health, that an interdisciplinary framework is desirable in public health and especially when the health service system is subjected to critical scrutiny (Nayar, 1993). However, it is necessary to understand the different theoretical and empirical levels which exist in such a framework.

The first level is to consider health (ill-health to be specific) as a problem that needs to be resolved. The purpose is to understand the nature and cause or distribution and determinants of diseases. In other words, the epidemiology of diseases forms the basis for an understanding at this level. The analysis of health problems in a society requires consideration of not only the growth of productive forces but also the level of inequality in terms of class, caste, and other social categories, gender, generational, and geographical factors.

At the second level, health has to be considered as a need to alleviate the suffering due to health problems. It is here that the analysis of social, psychological, and cultural factors is needed. Human beings encounter health problems when they interact with each other in a given social structure, in addition to when they interact with the parasite and the ecological context in which they live and work. The analysis of institutional factors including appropriate financing strategies for optimum impact of health policies have to be considered in this context. Non-accessibility and non-availability of health services to the people have to be explained not only in social, psychological, and cultural terms but in terms of the political economy as well.

At the third level is the international domain where the focus has to be on the imbalances in the world system which sustains poverty and inequality in individual countries. With regard to health, the influence of international policies in shaping endogenous actions and programs needs to be understood. Implementation of selective primary health care, tuberculosis program based on the DOTS strategy, and the pulse polio program are examples which show the ideological dominance of a public health strategy emanating from funding agencies located in the industrialized countries.

It is necessary to state that the three levels are in many ways overlapping and inter-related at both theoretical and empirical domains. This theoretical framework highlights the need to adopt a political economy approach as against segmented disciplinary approaches which are in vogue in public health. For instance, in the present understanding of social determinants in health, holistic views are based on a systemic understanding especially with regard to interactions between people and the health service system.

The political economy tradition which is subsumed in critical public health tries to locate the ill-health and health inequalities in a wider framework contextualized within the structure of the society (Mykhalovskiy, 2004). The political economy approach in health starts with a critique of the organization of the economy and the process of changes and their implications for the health of the people (Navarro, 1976). These critiques largely located their perspective arguments on a wider notion of inequality prevailing in the developing and developed countries, inequitable relationships within and between countries, etc. However, it may not be correct to say that political economy approach is only a macro-critique of public health trends emerging from societal restructuring and therefore theoretical, but even understandin of social determinants can form the empirical base for the approach. The fi for the political economy critique comes from the knowledge of pathway ill-health such as class and other social categories, inequality research The political economy approach therefore has to constantly undertake checks to develop its perspective analysis. For instance, the roles of d economies, the political traditions within these economies, and th framework which impact on health have empirical explorations framework (Navarro and Shi, 2001). One of the earliest empirical explorations influenced by a political economy approach is an ethnographic study on the introduction of Western medicine in Tamil Nadu, India by adopting a theoretical perspective which considers health not only a socially defined entity but also as a socially produced reality (Djurfeldt and Lindberg, 1976). The holistic approach considers social determinants from the point of view of praxis where the starting point is the perspective which is linked to trends observed empirically. The approach is valuable from the point of view of policy directions and functions as a barometer for large scale deviations in structure of the society which impact on the health and well-being of the population.

The reemergence of the social determinants framework in recent times has to be seen with this political economy approach. It is a challenge to the economic framework which came to dominate public health since the nineties after many countries in the South came under the structural adjustment programs. It is now realized that a dominant economic approach to health may not be realistic given the social fabric in societies which impinge on health and it is possible to say that the golden age of macro-economics of health is fading (Bhattacharya, Messenger and Overy, 2010). However, the current approach to social determinants is also overtly medicalized with the medical discourse and the medicine men channeling the social stream. This medical gaze results in the social agenda being too narrow and often addressing only the easier downstream or proximal options. Such dichotomous conceptualizations rather than a multilevel approach result in easier to manage proximal options (Krieger, 2008). "Class and racial inequality, for example, differentially affect the living standards, working conditions, and environmental exposures of the dominant and subordinated classes and racial/ethnic groups, thereby creating class and racial/ethnic health disparities. Stated more generally, a society's economic, political, and social relationships affect both how people live and their ecologic context, and, in doing so, shape patterns of ...ease distribution. The understanding of the societal distributions of health ...nnot be divorced from considerations of political economy and politi...y" (Krieger, 2008:223).

...lso considered as quantitative/demographic entities in a health ...pective with a framework devoid of embodiment extremely ...ch examines the interface between ill-health/body, the ...ate the conditions of ill-health, and the society. To ...r for the health systems/services development, ...onsisting of biological entities as sick in... ...consisting of the society, the institution ...ogy (Krieger, 2001; Krieger, 2005). Much ...ing the disorder that we discern and theorize ...e neglect of this eco-social dynamics.

An approach to health system and health service system needs to have a political economy framework which examines social factors and other distal factors contributing to health service development and health improvement. The way health systems and services are financed, designed, and delivered also acts as a powerful determinant of health (Doherty and Gilson, 2006). The interaction between health services and the people occur in a social context and it continually impinges on the way health services develop in this country. Health services can reinforce preexisting social stratification and also impoverish people. Many features of the health services such as resource allocation, strategies, priority setting, human resources, management, regulation, etc. have implications for ensuring equity-oriented health policy and service. Health policy analysis is a complex task rightly described as a 'beast' probably because it takes different shapes in different contexts and the dimensions are unmanageable and atypical (Walt et al., 2008). There are new actors and new mechanisms that are evolving in health policy and health system environment which need to be contextualized and deconstructed. It is for these reasons that a delineation of the factors which influence health services development in the country can provide insights for channeling it to develop an appropriate health policy environment.

OUTLINE OF THE BOOK

Anchored on the above-stated perspective, there are two fundamental themes delineated in this book which can be called as the main actors with respect to health services development in this country—the state and the civil society. The people who are the main respondents of health care are discussed as part of these two actors. This framework may be similar to the policy triangle framework which considers different actors who interact and shape policy-making (Walt et al., 2008). Closely interwoven with these basic themes are the sub-themes of policy cleavages (Hunter, 2008) and it may lead to some repetitive ideas or discussions. Argued in this book is the idea that the understanding of health service development in the country has been quite nebulous as it went through many ups and downs which have implications for making health and health services universal. This could be extremely important given the recent thrust on universal health care. This is the simpler part of the debate.

Such simple arguments although straightforward have to go beyond mere descriptions to capture the complexity. This is attempted in this book through an analytical synthesis of health service development in India. The book to some extent uses an iterative approach to reformulate, revise, and identify conceptual and operational levels involved while working in an interdisciplinary platform and in an academic domain. Many sections are based on analytical reviews and a few such as decentralization is based on fieldwork and interviews. The iteration depends on earlier papers written by the author. The book tries to decipher some of the essential domains of health services—the institution (mainly the state and to some extent the civil society), the delivery mechanisms, the policy changes and the people, and how they shaped the health services. It also tries to place these domains in the teleology toward disorder. Obviously, there is some disconnect, problems of presentation style, and the extant of description when these are presented in a book form and much depends on the way they are woven together. There could also be some repetitive statements and arguments which are unavoidable when the subsystems of the health system are deciphered in a discrete way. The important point is to recognize the interrelatedness of the components under discussion with the integrated whole i.e., health and health services. What could emerge from this critical discourse analysis is a thesis on how health services in the country are shaped or an understanding of the various actors in this process which result in a state of disorder. It may also provide some insights regarding the slow if not stagnant progress in achieving universal human health.

The theoretical position and a methodology of this book are revealed in this introductory chapter. The second chapter based on a critical reading of several government reports and documents (perhaps the most difficult part for the author and the reader!) attempts a historical analysis of how various committees constituted at various points of time have influenced the trajectory of health services in the country. The present ills with health services could be attributed partly to the bureaucratic approach adopted by the Indian state to deliver health services. This chapter enables us to contextualize the role of the state in a historical perspective. The present favor and fervor with privatization or public-private partnership emerge from such a historical context.

The third chapter deals with reforms and their various combinations. This is the process which can be appositely called "enzymatic"—a process in which the state actively takes intensive and proactive actions which result in digesting its role and encouraging the role(s) of other actor(s) such as private sector or NGOs or sometimes it wants to exert more control on the social processes through policies or legislations. The chapter gives material to understand the discourse, approaches, strategies, and the outcomes of reforms and is an expansion of the second chapter and therefore some repetitions are imminent. It was difficult to meander through the so-called cacophony of approaches, frameworks, programs, and projects which keep on changing. It is evident from the analysis that much of the reforms have had impacts which could be termed as below the optimum given the intensity in which the new approaches were driven.

From here onward, we move to the domains in which people are closely involved in the process of governance and decision-making. The much hyped decentralization initiatives in India which serve as the linkage with the state and the people are discussed in chapter 4. One can see the linkages between this chapter and the previous chapter on reforms. This chapter will especially examine the implications of decentralization for health services. The process of decentralization in India has been largely political although it is being instrumentalized in recent times as a part of the reform agenda. The conceptual and operational dimensions of decentralization with respect to health services have been analyzed in this chapter.

Chapter 5 discusses another dimension of the inter-phase between the state, civil society, and people. Historically, there was always intent on the part of the state to involve the civil society especially in the social sector. The process of delivering services to areas the state could not reach was delegated to NGOs and other so-called Third Sector Organizations. The recent addition to this domain is the Self-Help Group (SHG) which is the latest instrument to deliver the agenda set by the state and the international organizations and which fits very well into the neo-liberal agenda as well. The nuances with respect to these organizations are discussed in this chapter.

The final chapter offers a theoretical synthesis of the state of disorder and the possible teleology with respect to health services development. What could be deduced from the analysis undertaken in the earlier chapters is a process which can be called as homogenization of order through universal managerial and technical-biomedical interventions to restore the so-called order ignoring contextual factors. This chapter also highlights the interlocking nature of societal crises and the disorder in health services.

2

Grappling with Delivery of Health Care

A Historical Examination

The history of health services development in India was replete with many positive and negative trends and was influenced by a number of exogenous and endogenous factors at various points of time. Historically, apart from epidemiological, social, and economic factors, one of the important engines which drove the Indian health services was the bureaucratic decisions undertaken through committees largely dominated by generalists. This chapter delves into the essence of some of the salient committees which have shaped the health services in India by a critical reading of the recommendations and a reflection of the implications. Considerations of equity, coverage, epidemiological scenario, and the social and economic conditions of the people certainly played some roles in the initial blue printing of services. Based on our reading, we argue that the various milestones and the shifts that have taken place in health services development in India were influenced by international policy changes as well as their reflections on the various committees that were constituted by the Indian government periodically. Despite discontinuities, it is possible to observe that the bureaucratic and top-down decision-making and the strategies suggested by the committees could have indirectly helped the half-hearted transition toward a market-oriented health services or at least an Asiatic mode of market orientation in the social sector at present. The Asiatic mode of market orientation in the social sector is a cocktail version which retains the essence of neo-liberal strategies and which is a mix of public and private sectors with a reduced state control in the conventional sense but still highly bureaucratized. Decentralization is advocated but practiced only notionally. The National Rural Health Mission (NRHM) is an example of such an approach. Strategies such as public-private partnership, community based insurance, conditional cash transfer, promotion of self-help groups etc. represent the elements of such an orientation.

POST INDEPENDENT HEALTH SERVICE DELIVERY: A HISTORICAL ACCOUNT OF THE COMMITTEE APPROACH

The decision to use an allopathic system of medicine for the provision of health services in order to achieve a pan-Indian coverage was claimed to be the *modernizing approach* of the professional and political elite at the time of independence. The Bhore committee report laid the foundation of health services in the country with an extensive network of health institutions from the district hospital, the sub-district hospital (*taluk*), the primary health centers at the block-level, and the sub-centers at the village-level and it reflected the blueprint approach of the health planning and represented the first milestone in the health services development of the country. The recommendations of the Bhore committee were guided by "tendencies apparent in some of the more *progressive* countries of the world" (emphasis added). These included Great Britain, Australia, the United States, Canada, Soviet Union, and New Zealand. Among these, the health services prevalent in Great Britain, Australia, Soviet Union, and New Zealand had influenced the thinking of the Bhore committee (Government of India, 1946, Vol. 2:8-12). The committee noted that the medical care was very costly to large sections of the population in the United States and that the poorer sections lacked suitable medical facilities. The comprehensiveness of health services, which was the hallmark of Great Britain's health organization, was one of the principles adopted. It also noted that principles for the organization of health organization in Australia were also suitable for a country like India. These included—the right to health; the right to receive health care at the doorstep; the need to provide health care irrespective of the financial status. Similarly, the committee also took note of the system in New Zealand where the social security act stipulated complete and free medical service to the people. One could therefore consider this as the first exogenous influence on the shaping of health policy in the country.

However, the committee had some truly progressive visions despite the above orientations. The committee quoted Professor Henry Sigerist's following sentence to emphasize the need for universality, equity, and comprehensiveness of health care.

> Health is one of the goods of life to which man has a right; wherever this concept prevails the logical sequence is to make all measures for the protection and restoration of health accessible to all, free of charge; medicine like education

is then no longer a trade, it becomes a public function of the State. (Ibid., Vol. 2:10)

Thus, the "modern trend" according to the vision of the Bhore committee at that time was not only with respect to a model of health services and the use of allopathy as the system of medicine but also the provision of as comprehensive a health service as possible to the community and the coverage of largest possible proportion of the community. All the disease control programs have to be delivered by the state through the health institutions prescribed by the committee. This could be termed as a progressive public health vision. The Bhore committee proposed that in each village a health committee consisting of five to seven individuals should be established for procuring the active participation of the people in the health programs. This reflected the democratic vision of the Bhore committee which was largely ignored by the newly independent state despite a reiteration of the Gandhian ideal for *panchayati raj*. It is only since the implementation of the National Rural Health Mission in 2005 that something similar to this, like the Village Health and Sanitation Committee was evolved.

Generally, the Bhore committee favored a social insurance approach although by taking into consideration the conditions existing in the country it felt that the services should be free and the contribution from those who can afford to pay should be through general and local taxation (Government of India, 1946, Vol. 4:6). Interestingly, the committee proposed that governments of the future should decide whether the services could remain free or whether an insurance scheme could be introduced given the economic, social, and political requirements of the country at that time. This proposal of the committee is being realized, as at present the country is moving toward an insurance model for health financing after about six decades. The most important recommendation of the Bhore committee, which could be termed as the most progressive is: "no individual should fail to secure adequate medical care because of inability to pay for it" (Ibid., Vol. 2:17). Evidently, in recent times the government has shifted from this vision of the Bhore committee. The committee also recommended a whole-time salary service, which would enable the government to provide services in the rural areas where services are most needed. Thus the Bhore committee could be held partly responsible for the extremely bureaucratic and top-down health services as recommendations such as formation of health committees at the village level remained as finer points and were ignored. The committee also decided against the idea of a basic doctor with a shorter period of training and also against the indigenous practitioners which led to nonavailability of basic medical care to large sections of the population (Gautam and Shyamprasad, 2010).

The Sokhey committee, appointed by the Indian National Congress, endorsed the recommendations of the Bhore committee and also articulated the general conditions for the organization of health services (National Planning Committee, 1948). These were the "wasteful dichotomy" that has developed in the organization between curative and preventive activities; extreme poverty of the people and the inability to pay for medical care; and the availability of meager resources for care and research. The implications of such considerations were the need for an integrated approach to health services; free health care provided by the state; and optimum utilization of resources.

The Sokhey committee noted that although a number of ready-made schemes are available to provide health services to "modern communities," none of them was found to be viable for meeting the needs of the country or its resources. The health organization should be in tune with the features peculiar to India and should make use of the general principles outlined above. The committee also noted that given the extreme crunch in resources, there is a need to build the health organization in the cheapest manner possible and at the same time all-embracing which could take care of the health needs of the country. The committee mentioned, while endorsing the introduction of "scientific medicine" (*which meant Allopathic medicine*), that due to "appalling ignorance of the masses, and their religious and social prejudices," it is important to elicit maximum cooperation of the people by utilizing local talent to carry out the plan. A social engineering approach to modernize the "unmodernised" and traditional population is inherent in the philosophy of Sokhey committee.

The Mudaliar committee which came into existence in 1959 made a realistic assessment of the progress made in the implementation of the recommendations of the Bhore committee (Government of India, 1962). The committee noted that the primary health center program which developed did not resemble the one visualized by the Bhore committee, especially regarding coverage of the population. The Mudaliar committee, therefore suggested consolidation of the existing services than expansion and recommended that further opening of primary health centers be discontinued (especially without adequate facilities, resources, and personnel) until they are upgraded. However, the committee felt that this could be interpreted as a retrograde step, while at the same time recommending mobile vans for providing medical services to the rural population. It is surprising that even forty years after this recommendation, state governments in India such as Punjab are even now toying with the idea of mobile vans for providing health care to the rural masses.

The Mudaliar committee's vision was different from the Bhore committee although this was not clearly articulated in the recommendations. However, the intention to move away from a state-sponsored health care to an insurance based health care is again mentioned in the report. The committee suggested a long-range health insurance policy should be adopted by all citizens of India on the same basis. The rate of contribution however could be on the basis of the income of the persons concerned. The committee said that with regard to the *indigent* population, the state should continue to provide *all possible means* of health care. The committee argued for a distinction between those people who can pay and those who cannot pay for the services. The committee even considered an idea to introduce medical care cooperatives, another approach to move away from the state-funded health services. It is indeed interesting to note that since independence the state was inclined toward an insurance-based financing of health care in India and the present community-based insurance schemes are more or less similar to the one suggested by the Mudaliar committee.

The Chadha committee suggested that the basic health services should work in an integrated manner, which included family planning and other mass campaigns such as national malaria eradication program and small-pox eradication (Government of India, 1963). The committee suggested that multipurpose domiciliary services should be developed for all health programs including malaria, smallpox, control of other communicable diseases, health education, etc. The committee also suggested additional staff for polyvalent activities to make health services at the primary health centers and subcenters self-sufficient. Malaria was the overriding concern for the committee for suggesting organizational changes such as an extra medical officer at the primary health center or a malaria officer at the district level.

The committee, which was constituted subsequently known as the Mukerji committee, consisting of generalist administrators on the other hand, gave primacy to the family planning program and especially on organizational changes required for the Intra Uterine Contraceptive Device (IUCD) program. It suggested de-linking of malaria maintenance activities from family planning so that its staff could give *undivided attention to the latter* (Government of India, 1965). The most disturbing feature of the committee report is its emphasis on target-oriented approach and its method-oriented (IUCD) financial, organizational, and strategic recommendations for the health services. The target orientation was all pervasive, for the state, for each district, for each city, and for each block; it tinkered with the administrative system; changed the prioritization and undid the integrated vision which prevailed earlier. It is indeed surprising that just one method like IUCD which was discredited later could inflict so much damage to the health service system in the country. The influence of international organizations is quite discernible. The Mukerji committee has the following quotation of the World Bank mission:

> The numbers relating to various methods are impressive but the base population is so large that massive numbers of effective users are required if there is to be any measurable effect on the overall birth rate. (Ibid. 9)

This statement was used to advocate a vigorous, intensive, campaign-oriented, and paternalistic program to "tackle difficult areas and the resistant groups." This committee's recommendations had far-reaching implications not only for the family planning program but for the organization of health services in the country as well and could be called as the one which was partly responsible for the negative stereotyping of public sector health services in the country.

The committee which was constituted to look into the manpower, financial, and other requirements and the staffing pattern for organizing the basic health services with an integrated approach, in principle recommended an integrated approach to the entire health field. It felt that programs of public health and medical care should be integrated to the maximum extent possible. It also felt that an integrated organization should be developed at all levels of health organization and health workers should become multi-purpose workers. However, in operational terms, it came out with a preliminary and limited approach to "comprehensive" basic health care (Government of India, 1966). This basic health care purported to undertake only programs such as family planning, malaria, smallpox, health intelligence, and health education. Logically one could observe that there is no radical deviation from the method-specific approach advocated by the Mukerji committee. The committee, however, recognized close linkages between the pattern of basic health services, people's education, participation, and their socio-economic status. The committee assumed that as health conditions in the rural areas improve, the functions of the basic health services would diminish although even after about forty years, there are no remarkable changes in the health scenario.

The committee on integration of health services was constituted by the Directorate General of Health Services (unlike the earlier committees with the exception of the Chadha committee which were at the levels of Ministry of Health/Secretaries). The committee (known as the Jungalwalla committee) considered the philosophical and conceptual bases of integration at length (Government of India, 1967). According to the committee, the integrated health services will have: a unified approach for all problems instead of a segmented approach for different problems; medical care of the sick and conventional public health programs functioning under a single administrator and operated in a unified manner at all levels of hierarchy with due priority for each program obtaining at a point of time. Although the committee could not set out a concrete measure to achieve integration at the level of health programs, it did have some specific suggestions regarding organizational issues such as personnel and especially their pay and service conditions.

The idea of integration was taken forward by the committee on multi-purpose workers under health and family planning program (known as the

Kartar Singh committee). The committee (Government of India, 1973) felt that given the diverse, diffuse, and conflicting array of medical facilities, availability of such services to the underprivileged sections which constitute the vast majority of the population is inadequate. The committee noted that proper harnessing of the available resources and a reorganization of the entire system could help in solving the health problems of the country. The committee, like some of the earlier committees, also considered the question of malaria maintenance phase and small pox eradication apart from family planning program which all created vertical structures and staff and placed the issue of integration within this context. The committee, based on available studies and its own extensive discussions at various levels, recommended that given the extreme vertical nature of health services, it is desirable and feasible to have multi-purpose workers (both female and male) at the peripheral levels which it thought would enhance the acceptance and effectiveness of programs.

The report of the group on medical education and support manpower (Shrivastav committee) set a broader agenda for revamping health services from the primary to the tertiary levels and on reorientation of medical education as against some of the earlier committees which were examining specific interventions such as method specific interventions, cadre revision, etc. (Government of India, 1976). The report is relevant to understanding the emergence of a new agenda of community-centered health services (akin to self-help) taking shape in the late seventies. Although the present approach to self-help has been instrumentalized to a large extent under the neo-liberal strategy for a reduced role of the state and transferring of responsibilities to the individual and family, such an ideology was not discernible in the text of the report. However, intent towards a cocktail version of state-sponsored health care in combination with privatization and insurance strategies was present even at that point of time.

The committee apart from reiterating the need for developing an integrated service covering promotive, preventive, and curative aspects of health services and family planning and the importance of universal coverage and equal accessibility to all sections of the population also emphasized full utilization of para-professional resources and their supplementation by a well-structured system of referral services. The committee recognized that a universal and egalitarian program cannot happen in a social context riddled with mass poverty. It therefore underlined the need for giving highest priority and adequate allocation of resources for both health and education. The committee highlighted the individual, community, and above all the state responsibilities in health care. It thought that the overdependence on provision of health care through professional staff under state control had been counter-productive. It felt that this devalued the age-old tradition of community self-help and community autonomy and control over the provisioning of health care. It suggested a move toward self-help, creation of part-time semi-professional workers from the community itself who would be close to the people. They could provide promotive and preventive health care apart from basic medical services needed in day-to-day common illnesses which account for about 80 percent of all illnesses. This new system was meant for the "periphery" as the existing modern system was biased in favor of urban areas. This according to the committee implied creation of a health services within the community utilizing all local resources available, with a built-in referral services to supplement these activities. According to the committee, development of such resources starts with the family where the aptitude for health care starts and it believes that by appropriate educational programs the motivation for this could be strengthened. The committee visualized the following categories outside the existing cadre of health services (while being aware of its adverse reactions from the professional quarters and its negative implications in terms of letting loose half-baked quacks into the community) to emerge from the community:

- An adequate number of *dais* to perform maternity services.
- A large number of family planning workers from among adults, young men, housewives, and public administrators.
- Persons who will be able to provide some basic medical care from all systems of medicine.
- Persons who are trained to handle programs for the control of communicable diseases
- Persons who can help to develop promotional and preventive health activities especially related to nutrition, environmental sanitation, control of common diseases, yoga, etc.

The committee also suggested the creation of a National Referral Services Complex by developing proper linkages between the primary health centre and higher level referral and service centers. These were some of the general principles which the committee thought should guide the reorganization of health services in the country. It, no doubt, influenced the formulation of community health volunteer/guide scheme in 1977, modeled after the barefoot doctors' scheme in China which was later abandoned or disappeared.

The Indian Council of Social Science Research-Indian Council of Medical Research (ICSSR-ICMR) committee although not completely bureaucratically visualized and operationalized was set-up as a follow-up of the Alma Ata conference on Primary Health Care. It prepared a report on an alternative strategy on HEALTH FOR ALL, which also served as a precursor to the National Health Policy of 1983 (ICSSR-ICMR committee, 1980). The committee had a progressive vision (being outside the Ministry set-up) and it also had some continuity with the Shrivastav committee report in terms of its broad outlook. The report adopted a comprehensive definition of health and placed it in the context of socio-economic transformation (Nayar, 2012).

The committee recognized that the *existing health sector is exotic, top-down, elite-oriented, urban-based, centralized, and bureaucratic with over-emphasis on curative care*. It suggested an alternative model rooted in the community which could provide adequate, efficient, cost-effective, and equitable referral services; integrate promotive, preventive, and curative aspects; and combine valuable elements in our culture and tradition with the best elements of the Western system. The report suggested:

- integrated plans for health and development including family planning.
- reorientation of existing priorities so that the bulk of the funds can be spent on (a) programs on nutrition, improvement of environment, immunization, and education rather than on curative services (b) on basic community services at the bottom than super-specialties at the top.
- replacement of the existing model of health care with an alternative model which integrated promotive, preventive, and curative services and is community-based, participatory, decentralized, and democratic.

Despite a strong pressure to change the direction of the health services in the country, all the negative trends that the ICSSR-ICMR committee noted continued to plague delivery of health care in this country. Critics consider that the report as an ineffective intellectual exercise as it refrained from analyzing the implications of social conflict and the character of the Indian state (Qadeer, 2011).

THE EROSION OF INTEGRATED AND COMPREHENSIVE HEALTH SERVICES

The eighties saw further erosion in the primary health care ideals and the broader vision for health services. It started with a national health policy of 1983, which selectively picked up points from the ICSSR-ICMR committee such as integrated preventive, promotive, and rehabilitative services, health education, and some specific program while advancing the agenda of population stabilization, privatization, etc. The policy gave indication to the impending privatization plans of the government and to the reduction of government expenditure in the health field when it stated that private medical professionals and non-governmental agencies be allowed to establish curative centers and offered to provide logistical, financial, and technical support to voluntary agencies. The 1983 health policy also states that specialty and super-specialty hospitals in the private sector should be established which are integrated to the government primary health care system (Government of India, 1983a). According to the policy, private investments in the health sector should be sought to reduce government expenditure for setting-up such centers. It, therefore, redefined the recommendations of the Shrivastav committee on *referral services complex* by making the higher levels under the private sector. The intention to privatize, government health care system and to gradually withdraw from the health sector was implicit. From the 9th plan onward, there is a move toward the reorganization of health services with explicit stated intentions toward privatization, individual-family orientation, etc. The stated intention of keeping the health services available and accessible to the masses still found a place in plan documents but only as a mere opening ritual. The policy guidelines clearly showed the influence of the international donor agenda. The latter policy instruments, approaches, and programs in the new millennium were clearly influenced by these historical trends and could be called as the amalgamation of the continuities and discontinuities that were present at various milestones. Some of them such as the creation of uni-purpose workers were clearly positive while continued emphasis on vertical programs, intensive drives, introduction of user fees, public private partnership, etc. was retrograde.

During the early and mid-eighties, there were also further changes in the organization of primary health center network. The structure of district health system changed toward a more curative orientation by developing another institution called community health centers with specialists such as surgeon, physician, obstetrician and gynecologist, and pediatrician as well as three general duty medical officers from public health, anesthesia, and indigenous system of medicine (Government of India, 1983b). The staff pattern also included eight nurses, two pharmacists, two laboratory technicians, one X-ray technician, one extension educator, one ophthalmic assistant, one statistical assistant, sixteen ward staff, and ten supporting staff.

That mere availability of health centers does not always lead to better utilization is evident from the Planning Commission's evaluation study on functioning of the community health centers (Government of India, 1999). The community health centers (CHCs) were established as referral centers with the objective of minimizing the hardships of the rural people for accessing the specialized medical services available at the district and other referral hospitals, which are overcrowded. The study conducted in 16 districts of eight states shows that only two out of the 31 sample CHCs were used as referral centers. Eleven CHCs have not attended any referral cases while 18 have been used sub-optimally. The study also brings out that factors other than physical facilities are largely responsible for the suboptimal functioning of the CHCs. A comparison of the availability of staff and facilities in the thirty-one sample CHCs with their prescribed norms shows wide gaps. Most of them are not equipped to deliver the intended specialized services. More than 70 percent of the centers are running with either one specialist or without any specialist. The shortfall of specialists as against the required number was 74 percent in the case of surgeons, 61 percent in the case of gynecologists, 80 percent in the case of physicians, and 64 percent in the case of pediatricians. The most striking feature was the mismatch between the medical specialists and the corresponding equipment and staff. For instance, twenty-six CHCs had forty-two lab technicians, nineteen CHCs had twenty X-ray machines, eighteen had twenty radiographers, etc.

The most important finding of the study is that utilization of health centers was influenced by the ability to deliver the complete package of services. Variation in the availability of specialists, para-medical staff, and facilities for medical investigations, physical infrastructure, and the non-complementary nature of these inputs were found to be responsible for the differential utilization rates. The study points out that non-availability of one or more elements in this package could affect the utilization rates.

It is significant that despite all the constraints in the existing delivery system, a large majority of the households in the sample expressed their strong preference for public health care system as against the private facilities. Only about 11 percent of beneficiaries were dissatisfied with all the services of the centers in the eight states, while around 43 percent were satisfied with the services, another 45 percent were partly satisfied. The dissatisfaction was largely because of non-availability of medicines or lack of proper attention. The study also suggested that there exists an adequate demand of services from the community health centers. It is evident from the experiences of curative and referral institutions like the community health centers that it is not yet the end of the road for the public sector curative health services in the country and that improvement in the services can be affected through policy changes and systematic social and epidemiological approaches. This is especially important as the poor state of public sector curative institutions is used as a rationale for ushering in privatization in the health sector.

The same preference for public sector health services was also evident in another study on the primary health centers (PHCs) assisted under the social safety net program in Haryana, Orissa, and Uttar Pradesh (Government of India, 2001a). Despite a strong preference for government health care, they were not able to deliver services due to non-availability of medical and para-medical staff. For instance, female doctors were not available in many of the assisted PHCs. The facilities in PHCs have been created thinly and in an isolated manner as against the envisaged plan of creation of a complete package of complementary facilities in PHCs for facilitating institutional deliveries.

According to the 9th plan document, the suboptimal functioning of existing health care institutions is responsible for the non-availability of health services rather than mere availability of health centers (Government of India, 2004). Inappropriate location, poor access, lack of maintenance, lack of professional and para-professional staff at critical posts, mismatch between the requirement and availability of health professionals especially doctors at primary health centers (PHCs), lack of funds for essential drugs, lack of first referral units as linkage for referral services, etc., have been mentioned as reasons for the suboptimal functioning of primary care institutions. Taking cognizance of the widening disparities in the states in the availability of basic minimum services the conference of chief ministers in 1996 recommended that additional central assistance may be provided to the states for correcting the existing gaps in the provision of seven basic minimum services. But it is doubtful whether the pattern of utilization of such assistance could have led to any reduction in the disparities. This could be attributed to a diversion of funds by some critical states. Construction of buildings rather than improving the quality of services was given priority. Even the funds received from the department of family welfare and the externally assisted projects were used for construction of buildings. Thus the reasons stated by the approach paper for the suboptimal functioning of primary health institutions are only partially addressed. Apart from HIV/AIDS, non-communicable diseases also receive considerable attention in the 9th plan while diseases of the poor such as cholera and diarrheal diseases are ignored. It gives added emphasis on diagnosis and management through secondary and tertiary care institutions assuming that diseases like diabetes, cardio and cerebro vascular diseases, and malignancies are going to comprise the major disease burden in the rural areas. In reality, this could add to the program burden of the PHCs and community health centers (CHCs) and would also serve as a conduit for private diagnostic institutions sprouting up in the rural areas. The approach paper for the 10th five year plan (Government of India, 2001b) purports to review global and Indian experience in risk pooling, social insurance, individual insurance, health maintenance organization, etc. The paper also suggests that appropriate mechanisms should be explored for meeting the cost of serious illness and hospitalization by individual/organization and the state.

From the 9th plan onward, there is a move towards the reorganization of health services with explicit stated intentions towards privatization, individual-family orientation, etc. The ideals of the Bhore committee still find a place in plan documents but only as a mere opening ritual. The policy guidelines clearly show the influence of the international donor agenda.

The India Vision report prepared by the Planning Commission defines the criteria for more equitable and effective health services (Government of India, 2002a). These include:

- Universal access and access to an adequate level of health care without financial burden.
- Fair distribution of financial costs for access and fair distribution of burden in rational care and capacity.
- Ensuring that providers have the competence, empathy, and accountability for delivering quality care and for effective use of relevant research.
- Special attention to vulnerable groups such as women, children, the disabled, and the aged.

The approach to achieve equitable delivery of services is not envisioned clearly. The vision however gives an indication of things to come when it supports health insurance. It believes that health insurance can play an invaluable role in improving the overall health care system even to the levels of *panchayats*. The vision says, "the insurable population in India has been assessed at 250 million and this number will increase rapidly in the coming two decades. This should be supplemented by innovative insurance products and programs by *panchayats* with reinsurance backup by companies and government to extend coverage to much larger sections of the population" (Ibid.: 55). During the 11th plan period, the main thrust was on taking the limited role of the state forward by largely relying on quasi-state organizations such as state and district societies for the implementation of the National Rural Health Mission and trying out softer elements of neo-liberal instruments such as conditional cash transfer, contracting-out services, hiring of private specialists, community-based insurance, etc.

The report of the National Commission on Macroeconomics and Health is also significant in highlighting the need for increasing the investment in the health sector (Government of India, 2005). This is to be achieved:

> by increasing, widening and deepening the scope for taxation; increasing and strategizing deployment of donor aid for better outcomes; accrue savings by bringing in systemic organizational and financial reform aimed at optimizing resource use, reducing the flab and enabling a more efficient use of resources in other sectors as well; levy user fees on discretionary services at all facilities but within a policy framework that protects the poor through exemptions and concurrent monitoring of utilization of services by these groups, and/or insurance systems. (Ibid.:11)

The commission also has a simplistic oft-repeated neo-classical model on the health-wealth nexus existing in a two way process as a desired state. The neo-classical bias is quite evident when the report states that "healthier workers are likely to be more productive; and healthier children more likely to exhibit better cognitive skills, and become healthier adults" (Ibid.:21-22). The report, however has correctly diagnosed the factors which impede the functioning of health services in India. These include: weak management (such as poor management of resources and centralized decision-making, low budgets, irregular supplies, large-scale absenteeism, corruption, absence of performance-based monitoring, and conflicting job roles making accountability problematic); dominance of centrally evolved vertical programs which lack focus; absence of decentralization in decision-making in health services; selective-fragmented strategies and lack of accountability, etc.

It is evident that the so-called modernization agenda of the Indian state has resulted in a lopsided development of health services. The dichotomies it created could be multi-level. Apart from the sharp rural-urban dichotomies with regard to availability of the so-called modern health care which the state is trying to rectify through the implementation of special missions such as the National Rural Health Mission (NRHM) and also by experimenting with new forms of financing strategies, it also led to sharp division between allopathy and the Indian systems of medicine which the Indian state tried to rectify in recent times with the creation of a separate department for the same. However, the state patronage for allopathy continued to deny a fair deal for other systems of medicine in terms of budgetary provisions and institutional and political support despite accommodation of AYUSH (Ayurveda, Yoga, Naturopathy, Unani, Sidha, and Homeopathy) in the NRHM.

While, the shift toward newer ways of delivering health care such as introduction of insurance, and outright privatization of the health sector has not succeeded due to political pressure such as fear of losing people's mandate or due to popular protests, health in recent years has become a "soft target" for the introduction of such reforms such as a positive policy intent on privatization and introduction of managerial, individual-centered, and value for money approaches. The implications of neo-liberal packages will be extremely disastrous especially for the poorer sections as even with government funding, several constraints related to accessibility and availability of health care could emerge.

MOVES TOWARD PRIVATIZATION

Privatization of health care was an active agenda of the state in India although one could observe different combinations and levels of privatization in policy papers. The Mudaliar committee as early as 1961 felt that if suitable standards in medical care had to be established, public hospitals should levy fees for the services rendered both for in-patient and out-patient care. It also explored the possibility of promoting a medical insurance scheme while also supporting the development of medical care facilities on co-operative lines through suitable subsidies. Despite clear policy shift toward privatization in the National Health Policy of 1983, the 6th and 7th plan still echoed the minimum needs strategy and provision of health care through an integrated system involving primary, secondary and tertiary levels. It was in the 8th plan that references to privatization was made especially for secondary and tertiary hospital care.

The 9th and the 10th plans are more explicit on the issue of privatization. The 9th plan gives an added thrust to privatization of secondary and tertiary care institutions. A whole lot of concessions such as land, water, and electricity, and exemption of import duty for diagnostic equipment for the private sector are suggested for setting up tertiary care/super-specialty institutions. It appears that the government has only one pill of privatization under the World Bank medicine. The 10th plan admits that growing commercialization of health care and medical education over the last two decades has eroded the commitment to provide integrated curative and preventive care, adversely affecting the quality of care, trust, and rapport between health care seekers and providers. Having said this, the 10th plan also intends to explore different ways of health care financing including health insurance so that essential, need based, and affordable health care is available to all. The plan also purports to improve the efficiency of the existing health care system in the government, private and voluntary sectors, and building up appropriate linkages between them. Apart from this, the plan intends to increase the involvement of private, voluntary organizations and self-help groups for improving the access to health services (Government of India, 2002).

The National Health Policy of 2002 welcomed the participation of the private sector in all areas of health services viz. primary, secondary, and tertiary services (Government of India, 2002b). Both the plan documents and the health policy show a clear shift from the earlier cautious approach to privatization. The policy however, expects taking into consideration the past behavior of the private sector that its involvement will be substantial in urban primary and tertiary sector and moderate in secondary sector also envisages the co-option of the non-governmental practitioners in the national disease control programs

There is an increasing trend among the central and state governments to involve the private sector in public goals such as health and education. As evident in various plan documents reviewed in this chapter, the government at the center is keen to encourage this especially in the tertiary health care with a view to reduce government expenditure. The Public Private Partnerships (PPP) has emerged as a favorable option in states like Punjab, Delhi, Rajastan, Andhra Pradesh, etc. (Bhatt, 2000). The experience in some of the states however was not encouraging. The implications of having two different services, one private and the other public would further erode the quality of services in the public thereby aggravating the problems of the poor (Bhatt, 2000). This could also lead to disparity between the two sectors leading to migration of personnel, lowering of skills in the public sector, further cutbacks in the allocations by the government, etc. (see chapter 3 as well for recent trends).

The government, as evident from the national health policy, suggested the setting up of private insurance instruments for increasing the scope of the coverage of the secondary and tertiary sector under private health insurance packages. At the same time, it also toyed with the idea of introducing a health insurance system for the poor funded by the government but delivered through the private sector. This was considered as an appropriate alternative to an exclusive government mechanism to provide health services to the poorer sections. As a first step, the national policy suggested to introduce a pilot scheme in a limited number of representative districts, to determine the administrative features of the insurance model and to estimate the required resources. The results obtained from these pilot projects were utilized to evolve a national health insurance program what is now called as Rashtriya Swasthya Bima Yojana—RSBY (see chapter 3 for a detailed discussion). The Bhore committee's suggestion of considering insurance as a possible option at the time of independence has now become a reality.

PROBLEMS AND PROSPECTS OF INDIA'S HEALTH SERVICE SYSTEM: THE MANAGERIAL PHASE

There is no doubt that the health services in India are in a flux. The roots of the health service system have to a large extent been uprooted and the offshoots do not appear to be flourishing. The epidemiological and integrated vision at the time of independence has given way to a market-oriented approach. The half a century or more has also witnessed a number of changes in the organization of health services, most of them concentrated during the last one decade or less. The reasons for this new thinking is quite apparent, the influence of the World Bank during the post structural adjustment period and the reforms which were part of this package apart from a pliability of the ruling classes toward such moves.

It is possible to discern a consistent disdain for the public health sector painting it as a villain responsible for the poor state of health in India. This view is articulated not only in academic writings or the writings of independent scholars but it is reflected in many plan documents that we reviewed in this book. This view sometimes floated around based on some empirical studies as evidence is used as a rationale for privatizing health care or in suggesting other ways of delivering health care such as co-operatives, insurance, etc. The rationale for the poor performance of the government health sector needs some close examination before we suggest privatization of services. This will help in understanding the "evidence base" of privatization logic.

A few studies on the health services system in the country and especially on the primary care institutions reveal the overwhelming preference of the people toward government health care. Banerji's study on the rural health services in India revealed that accessibility and availability of health care are mediated by structural issues such as institutional inadequacies and inefficiencies in the system and influenced by various social, political, and economic factors (Banerji, 1982). The study changed the current knowledge regarding health culture among the Indian population and the "victim blaming" trend among some social scientists. The Planning Commission study reviewed earlier in this chapter is another such study which finds incompleteness in the availability of services as the main reason for the underutilization. The logic of completeness in the package of services that was responsible for the differential utilization of community health centers could also be applied to the primary health centers as well.

The government has also given in to the pressure of international donor agencies to adopt what can be called as the "one by one approach" or the categorical approach that takes up disease eradication programs concentrating on one disease at a time. The Mudaliar committee had noted that the method of dealing with diseases individually through mass campaigns is not conducive to the organization of unified efforts needed for the promotion of total health care (Government of India, 1962). After pulse polio there were indications that the government will go for a measles immunization program. These costly drives are undertaken by mobilizing of the entire health service system leading to a neglect of all other programs including other immunizations. Implicitly it means that India is not capable of eradicating diseases through an integrated and complete package of primary health services. The community is also made to believe that this is the program that is going to save the lives of their children (Razum et. al, 2001).

The National Rural Health Mission (NRHM), one of the flagship programs of the government, is projected as another attempt to arrest the slide of public sector health services (see also chapter 3). But in this process it also introduced several approaches, assumptions, and packages which strengthened and consolidated the neo-liberal trends set in motion by the structural adjustment reforms. The focus on secondary care and the neglect of primary health centers under NRHM are misplaced and could lead to further inefficiencies in the organization of curative care, delivery of national health programs, etc. (Qadeer and Dasgupta, 2007). It also introduced management principles into public sector administration. The managerial phase of health services development could have led to some positive spin-offs although it is doubtful that they are sustainable.

MATERNAL AND CHILD HEALTH

Among the different packages that the NRHM flagged, the *Janani Suraksha Yojana* (JSY) is claimed to have made some impact on institutional deliveries. The *Janani Suraksha Yojana* (JSY) is an effort to bring the poor, excluded, and marginalized women closer to the health services system through a facilitatory and participatory approach with the objective of reducing maternal and neo-natal mortality. The Accredited Social Health Activists (ASHA) who are women from the same community under this program serve as the link to motivate and support the women. The JSY is a program which combines economic support and facilitatory approaches to enhance institutional deliveries in rural areas. Public health scholars have raised a number of issues with regard to the JSY. One controversy is with regard to the overemphasis on institutional deliveries given the long-term mistrust of government health services, the credibility gap and the caste, class, and gender bias when women access care (Jeffrey and Jeffrey, 2010). The other issue is with respect to the component of privatization which some public health scholars argue could lead to further weakening of public sector health services (Nayar, 1998). Many states have started contracting private sector doctors and private hospitals for the institutional deliveries. The third issue is with regard to the approach of conditional cash transfer and the argument that it is difficult to attribute cash transfer alone to positive outcomes (Lagarde, Haines and Palmer, 2009)). Despite such critiques, some states in India have introduced people-friendly and socially and culturally oriented innovations in the JSY program although these could be in the form of small steps.

The impacts of these initiatives are not measurable yet. But as evident from the responses of grass-root level workers elicited through our own field work, there are shifts in the way in which the health services are perceived by the people (Nayar, 2014). Availability of services has changed the negative perceptions of public sector services. Study findings indicate a huge increase in utilization of the JSY scheme. In order to reach the stated goal of 80 percent institutional deliveries, more capacity needs to be created in health systems to cater to this JSY-induced demand (Government of India, 2011d; UNICEF, 2009). Methodologically, it is necessary to state that the impact of the policy initiatives on addressing inclusion have to be seen in deductive terms. The measurable change is in terms of health indices, that is, Maternal Mortality Rate (MMR) and Infant Maternal Rate (IMR). However, it is possible to assume that such changes are due to the policy and program shifts focusing on the women below the poverty line who by and large belong to the under-privileged castes in India. Moreover, the strong linkage between such focused action and the reduction in inequity is evident from a larger share of JSY beneficiaries among the women accessing facility-based care for deliveries. This is found out both by the Common Review Mission as well as the UNFPA Concurrent Assessment.

The United Nations Fund for Population Activities (UNFPA) evaluation conducted in five states revealed considerable improvement in institutional deliveries (figure 2.1). Madhya Pradesh and Rajasthan which belong to the vulnerable states have recorded high institutional deliveries compared to the previous years.

Although such a trend has not led to a dramatic decline of MMR as reflected from the MMR figures released in 2011, the decline for the vulnerable states has been from 375 in 2004–2006 to 308 in 2007–2009—a decline of about 18 percent which can be called as significant (Government of India,

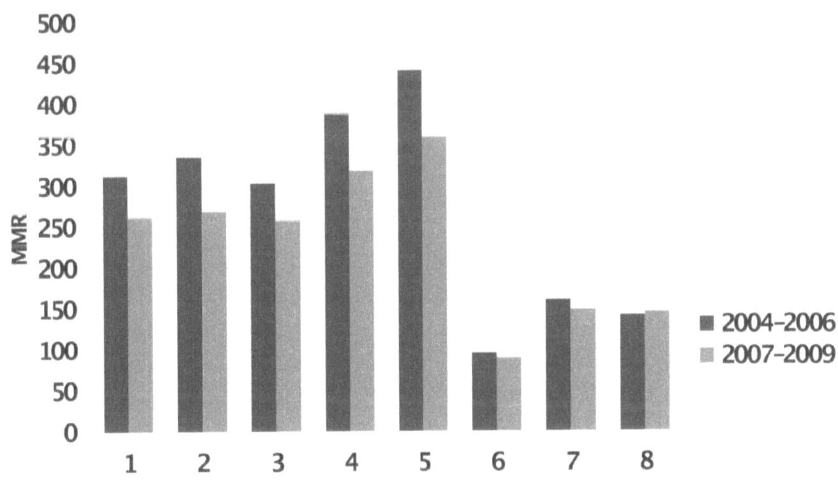

Figure 2.1. Trends in MMR in selected states 2004–6 and 2007–09
Source: Government of India, 2009a; Government of India, 2011a

2013). The all-India figure shows that MMR declined from 254 in 2004–2006 to 202 in 2007–2009, a fall of about 17 percent. Apart from Kerala, Tamil Nadu and Maharashtra have also joined the states which achieved the Millennium Development Goal (MDG target (Government of India, 2011a; Government of India, 2013). However, the linkage between high rates of institutional deliveries and MMR reductions is yet to be demonstrated.

MDG envisages reduction of IMR to 28 and Under Five Mortality Rate (U5MR) to 42 by the year 2015. IMR for the country has registered a decline of 3 points to 50 in 2009 from 53 in 2008. The maximum IMR has been reported in case of Madhya Pradesh (67) and the minimum for Kerala (12) (Government of India, 2013). Neo-Natal Mortality Rate (<29 days) and Post Neo-Natal Mortality Rate (1 month to 11 months) has declined by 1 point and 2 points respectively. Kerala (12) and Tamil Nadu (28) have already achieved the MDG target while Andhra Pradesh, Gujarat, Haryana, and West Bengal closer to achieving the target (Government of India, 2011a).

U5MR for the country has declined by 5 points over 2008 (64 in 2009 against 69 in 2008). A uniform decline of about 5 points is seen in male and female U5MRs. The maximum U5MR has been reported in Madhya Pradesh (89) and the minimum U5MR in Kerala (14). As of now, five states/UTs viz. Kerala (14), Tamil Nadu (33), Maharashtra (36), Delhi (37), and West Bengal (40) have achieved the MDG target (Government of India, 2011).

DLHS 2 and 3 data from 2002–2004 and 2007–2008 show that Orissa and West Bengal are the two states which have recorded considerable improvement with respect to antenatal checkups across different caste groups. Not only is there improvement in the figures in these two states, the social gap between different caste groups has reduced. However, in most other states, the effect of antenatal coverage was smaller. Other analyses based on NFHS rounds and DLHS also show that the states have moved to higher equity with respect to institutional deliveries (Shekhar and Ram, 2011). The linkage between cash assistance and increase in institutional care is evident from the increase in institutional deliveries especially in high-focus states like Madhya Pradesh, although this increase could be highly skewed and localized which is not reflected in the aggregate data. Preliminary analysis based on DLHS data shows that the JSY scheme has helped in the coverage of antenatal and intrapartum care and has also probably contributed to reductions in the numbers of perinatal and neonatal deaths although the effect on maternal mortality is not known (Lim et al., 2010). The uptake of JSY among the poorest and least-educated women has also not been high. The explanations for this trend are 1) the short duration of the JSY scheme, 2) problems in the physical access and, 3) cultural barriers against institutional births among certain groups (Lim et al., 2010). DLHS data also show that with respect to immunization coverage, there is considerable improvement in states such as Orissa, West Bengal, Chattisgarh, and Uttarakhand, especially among the SC/ST communities. The issue of whether the JSY could reduce inequities in care is still an open question which needs further studies (Das et al., 2011). For the moment, it is a matter of deduction that since coverage has increased as evident from the data the program could have led to some spin-offs in increasing access and acceptability of health services among the underprivileged sections in the country.

APPROACH TO NON-COMMUNICABLE AND COMMUNICABLE DISEASES

In order to control Non-Communicable Diseases, Ministry of Health and Family Welfare, launched the National Program on Prevention and Control of Diabetes, Cardiovascular diseases and Stroke (NPDCS) on January 8, 2008. The focus was on detection and awareness generation. A pilot project was launched in ten districts in ten states with health promotion and health education as the core activities. In July, 2010, the Cabinet Committee on Economic Affairs approved the National Program for Prevention and Control of Cancer, Diabetes, Cardiovascular Diseases and Stroke (NPCDCS) for implementation of its various components during the fag end of the 11th five-year plan (2010–2011& 2011–2012) at an estimated outlay of around Rs. 12 billion (Rs.5 billion for interventions on diabetes and cardiovascular diseases & stroke and Rs.7 billion for cancer control). The program was for implementation in 20,000 sub-centers and 700 community health centers (CHCs) in 100 districts across fifteen states and union territories by promoting healthy lifestyle through massive health education and mass media efforts at country level, opportunistic screening of persons above the age of thirty years, establishment of non-communicable disease (NCD) clinics at CHC and district level, development of trained manpower, and strengthening of tertiary level health facilities. Persons above thirty years and above are screened for diabetes and hypertension, early diagnosis of NCDs, and treatment at early stages. The pilot project could be the starting point for evolving a program focusing on behavior change in the community leading to adopt healthy lifestyles including dietary patterns, enhanced physical activity, and reduced intake of tobacco and alcohol resulting in overall reduction in the risk factors of common NCDs in the community (Krishnamurty, 2013).

The approach to the 12th plan, especially with respect to disease control programs gives an indication of the cocktailing process wherein the softer versions of the neo-liberal packages such as decentralization, community insurance, etc. will be mixed with a thrust on market-oriented diagnostics and curative care in the name of a changed epidemiological profile. Regarding non-communicable diseases (NCD), the approach continues to monetize the suffering in terms of money lost due to loss of lives. For instance, the approach paper for the 12th plan on non-communicable diseases states that India stands to lose 237 billion dollars during the decade 2005-2015 (Government of India, 2011b).

The approach paper on NCD gives the following suggestions:

1. Health promotion and prevention need to be given more attention to reduce the incidence of NCDs and their risk factors.
2. The states need to be given flexibility in implementation of the programs based on their public sector health system, prevalence and distribution of NCDs, and socio-cultural context. The flexibility would, however, be within broad policy framework.
3. Convergence and integration would be critical in implementation of a large number of interventions which would require unified management structure at various levels.
4. Integration of cross-cutting components like health promotion, prevention, screening of population, training, referral services, emergency medical services, public awareness program management, monitoring and evaluation, etc. would save on costs and make implementation more effective (Government of India, 2011b:10).

However, the quantum of investment proposed does not match with these experiences. The proposed budget in the 12th plan period is Rs. 580 billion which will be largely utilized for the following strategic actions (Ibid.:11):

- Health promotion for healthy lifestyles that preclude NCDs and their risk factors
- Specific prevention strategies which reduce exposure to risk factors
- Early diagnosis through periodic/opportunistic screening of population and better diagnostic facilities
- Infrastructure development and facilities required for management of NCDs
- Human resources and their capacity building for prevention and treatment of NCDs
- Establish emergency medical services with rapid referral systems to reduce disability and mortality due to NCDs
- Treatment and care of persons with NCDs including rehabilitation and palliative care

- Health legislation and population-based interventions through multi-sectoral approach for prevention of NCDs
- Building evidence for action through surveillance, monitoring, and research.

The mismatch between the experience-base, the strategies, and the budget is quite evident as the strategies will be largely concentrating on expensive and high-tech medicine rather than cost-effective preventive methods.

Although mental health also belongs to the list of non-communicable diseases, it has received special attention in recent times due to a vertical approach to disease control as well as its legal dimensions. Mental health, however, did not play any significant role in the health services development of the country. The National Mental Health program evolved only in 1982 although there are a number of initiatives since independence.

> These range from humanizing mental hospitals, moving the place of care from mental hospitals to general hospital psychiatry units, the formulation of the NMHP, adoption of the District Mental Health Program (DMHP) approach to integrate mental health with general healthcare, setting up of community treatment facilities, provision of support to families, the use of traditional systems of care, legislative revision, and public education and research to support the above initiatives. (Murthy, 2011: 100)

The National/District Mental Health Program (NMHP/DMHP) tried to integrate the mental health program with the general health care although this did not succeed as the entire emphasis was on curative rather than preventive services and lack of trained personnel hampered such an approach (Ibid.:101). The DMHP with a nodal status to a medical college was intended to take the program to the periphery. This also was ineffective due to a number of reasons such as lack of proper integration; limited capacities as mostly non-psychiatrists were involved in the program; lack of adequate monitoring; etc. (Ibid.:103).

The draft Mental Health Act of 2011 also is an effort "to provide access to mental health care and services for persons with mental illness and to protect, promote, and fulfill the rights of persons with mental illness during the delivery of mental health care and services" (Government of India, 2011: 6). It is supposed to supersede the earlier act of 1987 which is stated as not able to protect the rights of persons with mental illness and to promote access to mental health services. The act also provides for the formation of Mental Health Review commissions at the national and state levels. The move is toward legalizing psychiatric illnesses, which along with medicalization, could be detrimental to the persons with mental illness.

Health promotion is the major activity that could be envisaged as a cost-effective mechanism for non-communicable diseases. It is a challenging task in multi-religious and multi-ethnic societies riddled with many problems including poverty. The contradictions between stake holder interests and policies become very acute under such conditions. Considerable shifts in the health promotion and development efforts are needed in areas such as poverty and social justice, gender inequity, health and environment, control, and the changing epidemiological profile due to increase in non-communicable diseases (Mukopadhyay, 2007).

One of the notable health promotion activities undertaken in India by the voluntary sector is the *Khoj* program, the details of which are reproduced in box 2.1. This model can be used for wide-ranging problems including communicable and non-communicable diseases.

As against the approach to NCDs, the approach paper for the 12th plan to communicable diseases presents a different picture. The preamble appears to be extremely decontextulized with liberal mention of international data and regional experiences in an approach paper to the five-year plan of a country with such rich experience of controlling communicable diseases starting with tuberculosis. The neo-classical bias of stating productive years lost—a statement which continues to exist in all plan documents—is also evident in this approach paper. As stated in the report "the 12th Five Year Plan needs to address several public health challenges, such as ensuring primary health care to all including urban slum population, strengthening of health care infrastructure as per Indian Public Health Standards, increasing public health workforce, strengthening disease surveillance and response system, strengthening and networking of public health laboratories, optimizing use of modern information technology for disease control, formulation and enforcement of appropriate Public Health Laws, enhancement of public private partnership in disease prevention and control, increasing public health allocation and spending and decentralizing and communitizing planning and response" (Government of India, 2011c:17–18). The budget proposed is less than half of what is proposed for NCD, ie., Rs. 203 billion. Even admitting that grappling with NCDs requires a much more technologically oriented approach compared to infectious diseases, the approach needs a thorough debate with regard to its public health logic. It appears that a dichotomous approach to disease control and an extreme technology driven framework would only indirectly help the diagnostic, pharmaceutical, food, and information technology industries. What is needed in addressing public health challenges of the new millennium is an integrated vision and reiteration of the primary health care ideals in this third decade since Alma-Ata.

TEXTBOX 2.1. HEALTH PROMOTION PROJECT UNDER THE VOLUNTARY SECTOR IN INDIA

The Khoj project

- Khoj is one of the long-term initiatives of VHAI being implemented since 1993. Khoj, meaning search, has proven to be a successful model in the field of community health and development for improving the health status of the entire community through an integrated approach.
- The VHAI Khoj projects are located in some of the most remote and difficult areas with high mortality and morbidity rates, and where practically no semblance of health services existed. With a modest beginning of three projects in 1993, presently there are 22 such projects across the country in the remote pockets of various states such as Uttar Pradesh, Madhya Pradesh, Rajasthan, Bihar, Jharkhand, Orissa, Sikkim, Jammu & Kashmir, Arunachal Pradesh, Assam, Manipur, Tripura, and Nagaland.
- Direct health-related activities were given primary importance during the initial years and gradually, with improvement in the health patterns, other developmental activities were focused upon.
- The initial phase involved meetings with the district administration, health and education personnel, formation of village development committees (VDCs), identification of village health workers, capacity building of traditional birth attendants and periodic reviews of OPD clinics and mass health camps. Gradually, community organisation, income generation, women empowerment, non-formal education, and awareness generation became the main focus areas under KHOJ.
- Most of these projects are run by the village communities. These projects also successfully enhanced the knowledge, attitude, and practice of community members on health, nutrition, water, and sanitation.
- Khoj is basically an interface of health and other socio economic determinants and sectors.

Source: Mukhopadhyay (2007)

PROBLEMS OF NUTRITIONAL INADEQUACIES

There are already strong evidences from India that the total number of undernourished children has increased since 1990–1992 (Friel and Baker, 2009). Human development and poverty reduction need to be addressed with emphasis on nutrition as well. "Asymmetric economic growth, unequal improvements in daily living conditions, unequal distribution of technical developments and suppression of human rights have seen health inequities perpetuate and worsen, particularly over the last three decades. Addressing diet-related health inequities requires attention to the underlying structural drivers and inequities in conditions of daily living that disempower individuals, social groups and even nations from the pursuit of good nutrition and health. These are matters of economic and social policy at the global, regional and national level" (Ibid.:620).

In India, development of agriculture is strongly associated with the extent of malnutrition. As evident from a study, agricultural performance and productivity improvements seem to be critical indicating the need for interectoral action for nutrition (Gulati et al., 2012). There are a number of interventions such as the Integrated Child Development Scheme and the Mid-Day Meals Scheme (MDMS) for addressing the nutritional needs of children and women. "Other than these, relevant schemes include food-based safety nets such as the Food for Work Program under the National Rural Employment Scheme and state-specific schemes and initiatives. By the 1990s, the main initiatives to address nutritional security were via the food management system (buffer stocks and the Public Distribution System (PDS) network), food supplementation through the ICDS and MDMS, nutrition education through the Nutrition Board and ICDS, and health interventions to address the physical symptoms of malnutrition, micronutrient deficiencies, and maternal health" (Gulati et al.: 85). The Integrated Child Development Services (Supplementary Nutrition Program) under the Ministry of Women and Child Development provide immunization, supplemental nutrition, and early childhood education to infants and children up to six years of age, adolescent girls, new mothers, and women of reproductive age through centers for 1000 beneficiaries located in villages. This is an example of intersectoral collaboration between health and Women and Child Development which started in 1975. Given a number of weaknesses such as expansion of the program beyond the capacity, focus or emphasis on non-targeted population, and lack of adequate human power etc., a study in one of the poorest Indian states, Jhakhand, to evolve replicable low-cost strategy for involving community and family in child development (Dubowitz et al., 2007). The *community-based tracking* helped to reduce malnutrition in the study villages to a considerable extent.

What is required is an "ever green revolution" which ensures high productivity and nutrition security without associated ecological fallouts which was witnessed during the first phase of green revolution in India (Swaminathan and Bhawani, 2013).

Currently, there is huge debate among the scholars regarding the quantum of child undernutrition in the country. Pro-reformists would like to argue that there is exaggeration of stunting and undernutrition in the country due to the use of WHO global standards. This argument is advanced in order to justify the positive impact of reforms packages undertaken in the country (Panagariya, 2013). The counter arguments would focus on the multi-factorial and multidimensional genesis of the problem (Coffey et al., 2013).

> These include structural factors such as poverty; low status of women; poor public programs that result in distal and proximal factors like the inability of households to buy adequate quantity and quality of food; sub-optimal breast-feeding; inadequate frequency of infant and child feeding; and poor quality and low calorie density at each feed. Poor health of mothers during pregnancy results in low birth weights of about 30 percent of babies in India. Repeated infections, non-availability of safe drinking water, and poor sanitation are some of the factors that keep the cycle of malnutrition alive. (Gupta et. al, 2013:73)

Along with undernutrition, with upward mobility and migration to urban areas and with increasing mechanization, changing lifestyles and fast foods, obesity rates are on the rise resulting in dual nutrition burden-persistent undernutrition alongside emerging overnutrition. "This is a battle for minds, involving education, awareness building and persuasion, where no handouts or supplementation can help" (Gopalan, 2013:395). This current nutrition scenario has considerable implication for the disease scenario leading to dual disease burden of communicable and non-communicable diseases (Ramachandran, 2013). This then requires additional health policy impetus and fine-tuning of the health services which are already stretched to the limits and disordered.

HOUSING, WATER SUPPLY, AND SANITATION

Similar to nutrition, housing, water supply, and sanitation were sectors which were closely related to health and health outcomes but handled by other ministries such as Ministry of Housing and Urban Development, Ministry of Rural Development, Ministry of Drinking Water and Sanitation, etc. Environmental health, one of the sub-disciplines of public health, deals with "that aspect of public health which is concerned with those forms of life, substances, forces and conditions in the surroundings of human beings that may influence health and well-being" (Purdom, 1973). Housing, water supply, and sanitation form important components of the surroundings of human beings which influence health.

Housing

The blueprint with respect to independent India was evolved by the Bhore committee report and the sub-committee of the Indian National Congress known as Prabhavalkar committee report. The Prabhavalkar committee considered housing programs as part of the national plan and mainly urban-based (National Planning Committee, 1948b). It also suggested that no private players should be allowed in housing programs. With respect to rural areas, the committee suggested that housing programs should be part of the existing rural reconstruction schemes. The Bhore committee also considered housing as an essential public utility service and underlined the role of public utility service (Government of India, 1946). A rapid tour of India's five-year plan shows that the state housing strategies moved from aided self-help during the first plan period to a more subsidy-oriented program till the 7th plan (1985–1990). The most significant development prior to this period, especially with respect to rural housing, was the Minimum Needs Programs evolved during the 5th plan (1974–1979) which has housing as one of the vigorous activities to be undertaken. The Rural House site and House Construction Scheme formulated during the earlier plan period was strengthened during this period.

It was during the 7th plan that a major shift happened with the redefinition of the role of the state in house construction programs and reducing its role to that of a facilitator (Nayar, 1996). This role of the government being an enabler rather than a provider got further reinforced during subsequent plan periods with the entry of private players and the real estate sector. The housing program for the rural poor became more targeted with the *Indira Awas Yojana* for the Scheduled Castes-Scheduled Tribes and the free bonded labor.

The relationship between health and housing is more dialectical and complex which cannot be resolved by a reformist-welfare approach of provision of buildings. The experience of the One Lakh housing scheme in Kerala shows that an integrated approach with not just the provision of a structure only but the essential amenities such as electricity, water, roads, and culturally sensitive housing models as well could enhance the health effectiveness of the housing programs. A number of factors such as housing culture, housing behavior and perceptions, family formation patterns, spatial distribution of settlements which are region-specific, and nature of technology influence the housing programs in the country (Nayar, 1987). "Investment in housing can be more than an investment in bricks and mortar: It can also form a foundation for the future health and well-being of the population" (Shaw, 2004:397).

Water Supply

At the time of independence, only 12.7 million people in 253 towns in India had protected water supply. The Bhore committee recommended thirty-five years for complete coverage and as a follow-up several measures were undertaken. Prominent among them were the formation of an environmental hygiene committee in 1948 to discuss strategies and constraints with respect to hygiene and health including water supply. The National Water Supply and Sanitation Program with the assistance of USAID came into existence in 1954. A Public Health Engineering Organization also was created under Director General of Health Services which was later moved out to Ministry of Works and Housing.

The allocation in the first two plans was extremely meager with 80 million in the first plan and 840 million in the second plan with an urban emphasis. The major problem regarding planning of drinking water programs in India was lack of adequate data and the complexities in the availability and accessibility across the villages in India which fall in different socio-ecological zones. In order to collect relevant data for planning, the government appointed the National Water Supply and Sanitation Committee in 1960 (Nayar, 1996). The special investigation teams collected the data across the country which categorized India's villages into mainly three categories:

1. Those which do not have an assured source of drinking water within a reasonable distance of 1.6 km.
2. Those which are endemic to cholera, guinea worm, etc.
3. Those which have excess of salinity, iron, fluorides, or other toxic elements.

The first category of villages was called as scarcity and difficult villages and the second and third categories were named as health problem villages.

The main focus of the 4th five-year plan was on acute scarcity and health problem (endemic to water-borne diseases) villages. The survey identified 153,000 problem villages out of which 91,181 were acute scarcity villages, 33,857 cholera endemic, 3,184 guinea worm endemic, and 24,778 villages had water sources with risk from other water-borne diseases. (IV Plan

1969–1974.) An assessment was carried out during the same period which showed the following pattern:

Adequate with pollution risk	214,000
Inadequate unprotected	185,000
Problem villages	153,000
Adequate quality acceptable	63,855

The norms were also fixed for the provision of sources which was as follows in the beginning and were upwardly revised subsequently as the situation improved:

Rural areas

- 40 liters per capita per day-Lpcd (55 at present) within 1.6 k.m. or 100 mtrs. Height. (one source for 20 families/100 mtrs ht.)
- one hand pump for 250 households

Urban areas

- 125 liters per capita per day-Lpcd in towns with piped water and sewerage
- 70 Lpcd in towns with piped water but no sewerage
- 40 Lpcd for towns with stand-posts

The 5th plan (1974–1979) placed drinking water under the basic minimum need and the strategy to cover all scarcity and unsafe villages continued. The urban situation was slightly better in which only about 20 percent (1,229) out of 3,119 towns did not have protected water supply. The subsequent plan periods until the 9th plan did not change the strategy except the evolution of a drinking water mission in the 7th plan (1985–1990) and the formulation of Accelerated Rural Water Supply Program in the 8th plan (1991–1995) which was subsequently renamed as National Rural Drinking Water Program. This coincided with the United Nations International Decade for water supply and sanitation (1981–1990).

The mission mode and the reform agenda were further strengthened during the 8th and 9th plans when the Rajiv Gandhi National Drinking Water Mission was evolved. Significant developments during this period are adoption of the Maharashtra model in villages having piped supply involving strong community participation with village panchayat and water committee members being directly involved in construction and maintenance. The committee consisted of 50 percent women members and gave representation to the weaker sections. In villages with hand-pump-based supply, the Midanapore model was adopted with a water committee for each habitation and two women members as caretakers and Rs.500 for maintenance per hand pump and 50 paisa per family. The involvement of NGOs was also enhanced. The 9th plan envisaged complete coverage, sustainability, and surveillance but could not achieve the objectives. The 10th plan reiterated the same strategy and adopted the sector reform program which began in 1999. The state moved from provider to facilitator by transferring responsibility to PRIs and NGOs. The beneficiaries were made to bear the project costs on a cost-sharing basis and user fees were also charged.

One of the significant developments during the 11th plan was the Bharat Nirman program which adopted an integrated approach by identifying key sectors for development. This vision had a Health in All approach as well (see chapter 3). The 12th plan envisages further delegation of the responsibility to Village Water and Sanitation Committees. It also plans to enhance the sustainability, monitoring and surveillance, and maintenance of programs based on experience of such programs in several villages, Information Education and Communication systems, user charges, cost recovery etc. (Government of India, 2010a). Another new mantra of the reform process is water security which means—"Every rural person has adequate safe water for drinking, cooking and other domestic basic needs on a sustainable basis. Safe water should be readily and conveniently accessible at all times and in all situations" (WSP and Government of India, 2011:9). Cost recovery is one of the main strategies of the water security project as evident from the many lessons provided by the Water and Sanitation Program (WSP).

Compared to many programs in the social sector, the water supply program is a success story with an epidemiological approach to problem identification, village identification, and policy formulation. It is a fact that considerable increase with respect to coverage of villages with a drinking water source was achieved before the reform agenda took over with strategies such as user fees, cost recovery, delegation, etc.

Sanitation

The Water and Sanitation Program, an organizational initiative of the World Bank, considers the South Asian region as the hotspot where there exists the greatest sanitation challenges (Perez et al., 2012). More than one billion people worldwide lack access to any sanitation facilities and poor sanitation causes millions of people worldwide to contract fecal-borne diseases. In recent times, there are even efforts to consider open defecation (OD) and lack of sanitation and hygiene in India as powerful and persistent causes of undernutrition (Chambers and Medeazza, 2013). The high rates of ODs and high density of population are correlated with stunting in children. It is possible that faecally transmitted infections could have an effect on nutrition but this form of manufactured correlations can lead to techno-centric solutions which fail in a context riddled with a multitude of social and economic problems.

Sanitation did not take off as a major sector-based program in India largely due to lack of political will and the meager allocations in different plan periods, especially for rural sanitation. It was only in 1986 that the government initiated the first national program in sanitation known as Central Rural Sanitation Program (CRSP). The main emphasis of the program was on provisioning of community toilets, and building toilets in schools and primary health centers. The program failed to impact on coverage as it was based on the assumption that provision of latrines will increase its usage (SACOSAN, 2008). This has led to the formation of a new strategy known as the Total Sanitation Campaign informed by inputs from a global strategy evolved by the World Bank. The three components are creating demand, changing behaviors, and increasing supply of sanitary products. In 2007, the government of India issued new guidelines for the Total Sanitation Campaign (Government of India, 2007). The subsidy approach was withdrawn and the CRSP moved toward a new demand-driven approach.

The *Nirmal Bharat Abhiyan* (NBA) under the Ministry of Drinking Water and Sanitation is a comprehensive program with the new approach to eradicate open defecation by providing sanitary facilities in rural areas. The new approach focus on increasing demand from the community and enabling options based on their economic capacity by information education and communication, human resources development, and capacity development etc. Marketing of sanitary ware through rural marts known as sanitation marketing is also part of the strategy. In other words, sanitation has now become part of the global reform strategy with the responsibility completely shifted to households.

CONCLUDING OBSERVATIONS

A critical reading of the salient committee reports, government documents, studies, reviews, impact studies, and academic analysis undertaken in this chapter leads us to advance the argument that the newly independent Indian state was already predisposed to the basic tenets of the neo-liberal strategies such as insurance, privatization, transferring of responsibilities to the family and individuals, creation of self-help groups, etc. This was in combination with a dominantly neo-Malthusian tone and tenor in the committee reports including the Bhore committee which led to widespread negative stereotyping of health services in the country. Such a committee approach also led to the creation of a centralized service and a bureaucratic organization as well as overreliance on health services to achieve better health for the citizens. Secondly, it can also be surmised that the *exotic, top-down, elite-oriented, urban-based* health services in India as pointed out by the ICSSR-ICMR committee report resulted from such a policy inclination of the state. Evidently, such a policy climate enabled the easy ushering in of market-oriented reform process since the nineties although in a subtle and cocktail form.

It is time to recognize that the utter neglect of primary care and primary health care institutions has influenced utilization of health services and contributed to worsening epidemiological profile in the country (Nayar, 2000). Such recognition at various points of time has led to distress actions, missions, and packages. Cost-effective interventions such as rational distribution of financial and medical resources including drugs, effective manpower distribution and primary health care approaches are brushed aside for ushering in the privatization logic and business models. Highly intensive drives, techno-centric packages and vertical efforts and costly building activities that are being carried out by even using the external assistance given under the safety net programs rule the approach to health care today. The move toward privatization or similar packages in health as well as in sectors closely related to health such as housing, water supply, and sanitation clearly comes out of externally imposed conditionalities rather than an internally arrived consensus. From a scientific point of view, such logic does not have an "evidence base," a term which is often posed by the so-called protagonists of techno-managerial packages and concepts to those who believe in integrated and unified efforts. Most of these can be termed as "eminence based" where some committees of national and international experts and groups decide in the name of larger interests of the people.

3

Reforms and Their Forms in Health Services

The disordering of health services in India can be diagnosed as an outcome of the many reforms the health services has passed through since independence. The reform era during the post-nineties however is replete with many new trends in organizational strategies which require analysis from a political economy perspective. There are many gaps between the typical reform packages of international donor agencies and their actual operationalization in many countries although the essence and essentials of the packages get implemented.

We normally tend to consider reforms in relation to public management or administration as a neutral operation and changes needed to improve the efficiency and performance of larger systems delivering services to the people. In the history of health services development outlined in the previous chapter one could discern many such instances of "neutral operations." However, in recent years the new externally driven approach to reforms in public systems has gained notoriety given its ideological basis and conditionalities which sometimes go against justice and established norms of a welfare state. It is important to recognize the differences between internally driven reforms and the so-called imposed reforms which come as a package from international donors. It is evident that the authoritarian-imposed package with supposedly measurable inputs and outputs more often distort the holistic and integrated delivery of health services (Moore, 1996). They often lead to reductionist approaches with vertical-time bound programs as solutions.

In the backdrop of the two ways of reforms that are present in the health service development of India, there are a number of instances which could be termed as milestones. These milestones could be considered as internally motivated reforms intended to improve the efficiency and performance of the health services system.

Conversion of uni-purpose health workers into multi-purpose workers was one of the important reforms undertaken regarding the delivery of health services (see chapter 2). This reform measure was suggested to off-set the extreme verticalization and the conflicting array of medical services that was prevailing in the sixties and seventies. Especially, this was needed to neutralize the negative influence of family planning program on the comprehensiveness of health services. Unfortunately, such a bold and timely reform process did not have a beneficial impact on the health services as the system continued to be preoccupied with family planning activities and as the spirit of comprehensiveness was not inculcated among the multi-purpose workers. Gradually even the idea of creating a cadre of primary health workers was de-emphasized as most of the subsequent vacancies, especially of male multi-purpose workers, were left unfilled.

The creation of community health centers (CHCs) as the First Referral Units was a major milestone in the delivery of health services in the country. The main feature of an upgraded PHC or CHC is a 30-bedded hospital. The staffing pattern of a CHC is four specialists (surgeon, physician, obstetrician and gynecologist, and pediatrician); three general duty medical officers (public health, anesthesia, and one indigenous systems of medicine); eight nurses; two pharmacists; two laboratory technicians; one X-ray technician; one extension educator; one ophthalmic assistant; one statistical assistant; sixteen ward staff; and ten other supporting staff. The community health centers were established to reduce the hardships of the rural population for accessing specialist services but subsequent evaluations show that even the objective of providing a referral for curative care has not been achieved due to several problems (see chapter 2).

The Community Health Volunteer Scheme (CHV Scheme) is another major intervention in the history of health services development in the country to place people's health in the people's hands by having a representative of the community dealing with the basic health care in rural areas and serving as a link between the people. The scheme was inspired by the Chinese barefoot doctors' scheme and was implemented immediately after the Janata Party government came to power in 1977. The democratization of health services, the essence of the CHV program, could not succeed due to the extreme bureaucratization and professionalization that prevailed within the health services (Banerji, 1985). This was unfortunate as the opportunity for a reform during the post-Alma Ata period that would have given primacy to primary health care and the people was lost due to poor implementation. The priorities also got changed moving away from the basic tenets of primary health care such as curative action taking precedence over preventive and the individual action over collective action (Jobert, 1985).

The National Rural Health Mission is the latest reform measure in the health services of India largely influenced by an endogenous process and political compulsions to mollify the disenchanted voters. The key strategies of the Rural Health Mission include: ensuring intra- and inter-sectoral convergence, strengthening public health infrastructure, increased community ownership, village level cadre of health workers, public-private partnerships, emphasis on quality services, and enhanced program management inputs. The mission has also suggested certain concrete measures. For instance, intersectoral convergence is proposed to be achieved by establishing yet another organization, this time probably a quasi-government society at the state and district level. The public health infrastructure will be strengthened by several measures; a few of them would probably script the demise of the public sector. These include engagement of private doctors, health committees with the power to charge user fees, etc. The community participation will be enhanced by giving functional responsibilities and powers to the *panchayati* raj institutions apart from by the creation of a cadre of voluntary Accredited Social Health Activists (ASHA), creation of a drug and contraceptive depot at the village, etc.

We could observe that even the endogenously evolved reforms have slowly started absorbing the essence of exogenously driven reforms and have been adopting approaches such as public-private partnerships, privatization, etc. such as some of the propositions that we find in the National Rural Health Mission. It is important to understand the origin of these approaches—the new ideas and doctrines—in public services as well as their ideological underpinnings.

NEW IDEAS AND DOCTRINES

The new ideas and doctrines on organization of public services based on the *logic of planned markets* have largely come from donor agencies like the World Bank and the Asian Development Bank and specialized UN agencies like the World Health Organization. These are often couched in technical and management language which appeal to generalist administrators and are often thrown in as indicative options rather than prescriptions (Saltman, 1995). These are largely unquestioned assumptions based on certain strategic principles of the donor agencies. Most of the reforms are intended to make organizations more like firms operating in markets (Moore, 1996). These assumptions are based on the notion that developing countries lack the necessary infrastructural and managerial resources to deliver public services.

The New Public Management (NPM), an Anglo-American product, has been the core approach behind this move. The NPM essentially is a value-for-money approach which suits the donor agencies and it is known by different names such as modernizing government, management by objectives, etc. For the proponents of NPM, the reforms are intended to increase efficiency by improving input-output ratio within the public sector. It also purports to improve accountability and transparency within the system (Sigamani, 2005). Partnership is also a key word within the NPM strategy under which the main thrust will be public-private partnerships. One of the implicit objectives of NPM is to reduce political control of decision-making and increase the role of managers.

Some of the strategies under new reforms include downsizing by reducing the number of public sector employees by voluntary retirement (golden handshake); reduced recruitment of staff especially at the lower levels; increasing salary differentials between the high ranking and lower staff; restoring key elements of a traditional bureaucracy such as order, hierarchy, and accountability, etc. It also includes contract management by contracting out some key services to the private sector, creation of autonomous organizations such as health corporations and societies as in AIDS control, introduction of user charges, etc. Some of these measures have already been implemented in several states of India without adequate operational research or evidence base.

Generally, cost-sharing and risk-pooling initiatives had a negative impact on accessibility and utilization health services in poorer countries. The frequency of use of medical services decreased significantly almost everywhere after the implementation of cost-sharing measures such as user fees (Holst, 2006). There are abundant array of evidence, which shows that people with the highest need of medical services such as the poor and people suffering from communicable diseases could not afford out-of-pocket expenditure. User charges also affect the access of women and low-income groups to basic services. Clearly then, there is a need to rethink about the utility of these strategies in the delivery of health care in India. OECD and WHO advocate free primary-level services; free services for targeted groups or communities; free services for priority diseases or conditions; exemption systems for hospital services; charges for the use of tertiary care by those who can afford it (cited in Holst, 2006).

The Modernizing Government Program (MGP) strategy in Kerala initiated under the aegis of the Asian Development Bank is a strategy using poverty as a platform to usher in a fiscal reform process in a number of important sectors of the government (Asian Development Bank, 2002). The MGP particularly targets the profitable power sector and social sectors such as health and education to move toward a market orientation. The poverty reduction strategy on the other hand is by extending the self-help approach and enlarging credit mechanisms. The health services are also targeted by developing sustainable financing strategies such as standardizing health services, fixing charges for services at different levels, etc.

There are number of criticisms against the strategy of modernizing the government or the new public management (Moore, 1996). Some of these are:

- The difficulty in measuring outputs or outcomes in many public agencies such as health services.
- The implicit assumption of value for money on which the model is based leads to a notion that if governments can deliver services as economically as possible, then the standard is met. It ignores the standards of fairness and justice.
- It could empower private sector interests such as pharmaceutical companies, equipment suppliers, health care companies, and private medical practitioners to exercise considerable influence on policy decisions.

The new approach to public sector management and especially public sector health services is a near total deviation from the earlier administrative principles based on equity, equality, and epidemiology to one, which are market-driven aimed at gradual downsizing of public sector health services. What could be called as a "managerial perversion" which became much more pronounced during the NRHM phase of India's health service development could lead to distortion in the delivery both primary and secondary health care as warned by some scholars (Chase and Carr-Hill, 1994). This is also part of the package of shifts based on a social model of health to one based on an individual model of health. There is no doubt that this will create vast gaps and chasms within the population and demolish the democratic traditions in health services.

DEBATES AND DISCOURSES ON REFORMS

The health sector reform program which is a corollary to the structural adjustment program rationalizes a number of its actions based on the issues of inefficiency, spending on inappropriate and inefficient services, etc. It also questions the high component of salaries in the public sector compared to operating costs. It also laments that services are inaccessible and that services are unresponsive although they are over-staffed (Cassels, 1995).

The present reform process under the structural adjustment programs also has another rationale. It is apparently undertaken in response to a fiscal crisis.

Therefore, the various strategies are intended to enforce financial discipline. The first target of such financial disciplining strategies is the public sector. In order to reverse these trends, the health sector reforms have a number of components such as improving the performance of the civil service (as discussed in the previous section), decentralization (see chapter 4), improving the functioning of the national ministries of health through organizational restructuring, improving human and financial resource management, etc., broadening health financing options such as introduction of user fees, community financing, social insurance, etc., introduction of managed competition between providers, and working with the private sector (Cassels, 1995). In effect, however, what happens is not financial discipline but delegation and privatization of services delivered through the public sector. In the health services, this has serious implications, some of which have been discussed in a critical discourse evolved during the nineties and after (Qadeer, Sen, and Nayar, 2001).

WITHERING COMPREHENSIVE CARE

It is now well-known that the health reforms that we encounter at present are part of the global agenda that is linked to market and trade in a globalizing world (Sen, 2003). Health sector is now being considered as an area worth investing in order to reap profits. It is also recognized that such a capital investment may not be sustainable in areas where profits may not be forthcoming, i.e., in a comprehensive approach involving preventive and primary care as well. The 1993 World Development Report foresaw this while suggesting bifurcating preventive care for the state and curative care for the private sector and defined an essential clinical package (World Bank, 1993). Such bifurcation kills the spirit of comprehensiveness of health programs. In fact one of the essential features of the primary health care strategy has been this approach where there is recognition of linkages between preventive, promotive, curative, and rehabilitative care which are located in the overall development of the community.

GOALS AND TARGETS

The First Goal-setting: The Bhore Committee

As also discussed in chapter 2, the first goals for the Indian health services were suggested by the Bhore committee (1946); the recommendations of which laid the foundations of the health services in the country (Government of India, 1946). These included both short-term program for two five-year plan periods and a long-term program for a distant future. With respect to the primary units, the short-term goal was to set-up primary health centers with coverage of 40,000 each with secondary health center as a supervisory institution. In the long run, the committee visualized a PHC to serve a population of only 20,000. The functions of the PHC included curative care to both inpatients and outpatients, maternal and child health services including family planning, communicable diseases, school health, environmental sanitation, and health education. The Mudaliar committee appointed by the government of India in 1959 and which submitted its report in 1961 noted that the primary health center program bears no resemblance to that visualized by the Bhore committee (Government of India, 1961). The committee was of the view that it will not serve any useful purpose to open PHCs without adequate facilities, resources and personnel (Ibid.:116). It took more than three decades to achieve something distantly similar to the even short-term goals of the Bhore committee.

Targets and Their Failure in Family Planning

The fate of the family planning program is well-known which went through rough roads on a number of occasions. Adoption of a stringent control rather than welfare strategy, excessive use of coercion to achieve targets, use of methods with perceptible side-effects, thrusting targets on the personnel and disturbing the integrated working of the health services for intensive drives, etc. are all reasons which created a negative stereotype regarding the program. Failure in achieving the goals of NRR 1 could be attributed to the social determinants which the techno-centric program could not address.

The target-driven approach was only discontinued during the post-Cairo period and largely as a result of the RCH philosophy which advocated a target-free approach for the health workers.

Health For All by 2000

One of the most positive milestones as a policy and perhaps the most negative in terms of its outcome in international health, Health For All (HFA) and the primary health care (PHC) strategies had some major influences on the health services in different countries including India, at least at the level of policies. The joint report of the WHO/UNICEF presented at the conference can be considered as a treatise on social sciences in health although the essence of the report never got translated into concrete actions (WHO, 1978). The report does not see primary health care as a set of targeted actions or goals but rather as a comprehensive strategy to achieve Health For All. A health system is visualized as consisting of interrelated components from both health and other sectors. The goal of Health For All thus can be achieved only by comprehensive actions in coordination with overall development of the society, community participation, self-reliance, decentralization, and appropriate organizational strategies.

Government of India appointed a working group on health for all by 2000 AD which submitted its report in 1981. According to the report, Health For All included provision of a minimum package of health care services to all the segments of the population giving priority to the underprivileged sections of the society (Government of India, 1981). The package included:

- Health education concerning prevailing health problems and the methods of prevention and control
- Adequate food supply to improve nutritional status
- Protected water supply and sanitary facilities
- Provision of appropriate health care to vulnerable sections such as children and pregnant women including family planning
- Prevention of communicable and non-communicable diseases
- Access to essential medicines and medical care

Like the Millennium Development Goals, the report identified a number of indicators to be achieved by the year 2000. Evidently, the comprehensive strategy suggested by the WHO/UNICEF Report was largely ignored.

Let us look at the achievement as visualized by the report in this thirtieth year of the Alma Ata declaration. Table 3.1 shows that most of the projections of the Health For All (HFA) committee have not been met in 2000. Especially the maternal mortality rate is extremely high even in 2004. Similarly, the percentage of deliveries conducted by trained birth attendants and the natural growth rate is also considerably lower than that projected by the HFA committee. The poor track record of achieving goals is quite evident and it questions the very basis of target-setting in health care.

The Reproductive and Child Health program

The Reproductive and Child Health (RCH) program is an example of unrealistic setting of goals. The evaluation report of the RCH—I find that the project goals were over ambitious in relation to the time available. There was lack of clarity regarding activities which resulted in uni-focal actions. Although the project approach talked about reproductive health and gender equality, it focused more on female sterilization (Sharma, 2007).

Table 3.1. HFA projections and achievements (Projected/targeted figures of the HFA committee in parenthesis)

Index	1981 HFA report	1985	1990	2000	2004
CDR	14.1	11.8	9.7	8.5 (9)	7.5
CBR	33.2	32.9	30.2	25.8 (21)	24.1
IMR	129	97	80	68 (below 60)	58
MMR	800		570	540 (below 200)	301
Net Reproduction Rate	1.67	2.0	1.8	1.5 (1)	1.4
% of Deliveries by TBA	10–15	18.7	22.9	29.0 (100)	26.1
Life Expectancy	52.6 M 51.6 F	55.4 F 55.7 M	57.7 58.1 (58.0 57.7)	61.0 62.7 (64)	64.8 65.6 (2001–06)
Natural Growth Rate	1.9	2.11 (1.79)	2.05 (1.66)	1.73(1.26)	1.66

Sources: Government of India, 2008; Government of India, 2006a

It also adopted a uniform package across states without consulting the states and other agencies. It gave so much emphasis on the target-free approach which was not followed in many states. The lack of training on such an approach negatively affected the process of decentralized planning. Although the goal of 60 percent of the district plans being prepared in a decentralized manner was met although true community consultations was missing in many plans. One of the key goals of the RCH I was to reduce the disparities in RCH between the regions, socio-economic groups, etc. However, comparison of RHS data for EAG states for both the rounds of surveys (Bihar, Chhatisgarh, Jharkhand, Madhya Pradesh, Orissa, Rajasthan, Uttar Pradesh, Uttaranchal) indicate no reduction in disparities in RCH status. Especially with regard to antenatal care, institutional delivery, safe delivery, full immunization, etc. there is an increase in the gap between all India and the EAG states (see table 3.2). Despite this experience, the RCH II propose new goals such as increasing couple protection rate, antenatal and immunization coverage, maternal mortality, etc.

The history of goal-setting in India provides some valuable lessons for the health services development in the country. This suggests that the whole process of goal-setting has to be re-examined. The process has to be realistic based on the epidemiological pattern and the natural history of any specific problem. The reasons for the under achievements in programs evident from

Table 3.2. Goals and the Gap in RCH

Comparison of EAG States with All India Performance

	RHS I 1998–99		*RHS II^ 2002–03*		*Gap (India–EAG)*	
Indicator	*India (%)*	*EAG (%)*	*India (%)*	*EAG (%)*	*1998–99*	*2002–03*
CPR any Method	42.5	33.7	49.0	41.4	11.0	7.6
Unmet Need	25.3	31.6	18.6	21.9	–6.0	–3.3
Any ANC	65.3	52.7	77.2	62.7	12.6	14.5
Institutional Delivery	34.0	19.7	46.9	24.1	14.3	22.8
Safe Delivery	40.2	26.7	62.1	39.4	13.5	22.7
Full Immunization	54.2	41.8	49.5	36.6	12.4	12.9
Home Visit*	14.8	9.8	6.4	4.7	5.0	1.7

^ Based on 50% of districts covered in Phase I of Round II

* Any health worker during 3 months prior to survey

Source: Government of India, 2008

the above examples could be multi-dimensional. It indicates organizational weaknesses not just at the time of implementation as is often pointed out but even at the time of planning and programming itself. Failure in implementation could be the result of unrealism and lack of vision at the planning stage. It also means that the complexity of the problem cannot be tackled by targeted interventions based on aggregate data as targeted interventions could lead to techno-centric packages ignoring the larger structural dimensions of the problem. The target-driven programs can also result in intensive, vertical and categorical programs which may distort the comprehensiveness of health services as has happened with the attempt to eradicate polio. The target driven and time-bound approaches could also place unrealistic demands on the existing fragile and crumbling delivery systems in the developing countries.

Notwithstanding these critical dimensions related to goal-setting, more and more goals are being suggested such as grand challenges in global health by the Bill and Melinda Gates Foundation (Birn, 2005) and global challenges in non-communicable diseases. Without being ambiguous, one can state that the epidemiological profile globally has been changing, with a nebulous mix of communicable and non-communicable diseases (Daar et al., 2007). However, the questionable feature of these profiles is the estimates and relative weight of the two. Firstly, the word grand itself could be inappropriate when referring to disease and death (generally it means majestic, impressive, inspiring etc.) and such an adjective need not have been used when it was used by the Bill and Melinda Gates Foundation for global health It is not surprising that the grand challenges for global health being a technology driven program to control diseases which kill millions developed into a global program with liberal funding from the foundation (Singer et. al, 2007). However, the claim that non-communicable diseases claim more lives than infectious diseases needs much more sound data basis than just estimates. The second issue is with regard to the goals themselves. Even admitting that grappling with the diseases under reference requires a much more technologically oriented approach compared to infectious diseases, the approach need a thorough debate with regard to its public health logic. It appears that a dichotomous approach to disease control and an extremely technology driven framework would only indirectly help the diagnostic, pharmaceutical, food, and information technology industries. What is needed in addressing public health challenges of the new millennium is an integrated vision and reiteration of the primary health care ideals.

Emergence of Millennium Development Goals

The MDGs has abstracted the essence of the Millennium Declaration of the United Nations in eight specific and concrete actions to be completed by 2015: 1) eradication of extreme poverty and hunger, 2) universal primary education, 3) gender equality and empowerment of women, 4) reduction of child mortality, 5) improvement of maternal health, 6) combating HIV/AIDS, malaria and other diseases, 7) ensuring environmental sustainability, and 8) developing a global partnership for development. With such overemphasis on health, MDG is a culmination of a decade of efforts to target specific and selective actions, such as in malaria-TB-HIV/AIDS, reproductive health-sexual health, polio eradication, etc. and the entire "evidence-base" that was generated to support such targeted actions.

The goals of achieving reduction of mortality rate among children under five and the maternal mortality rate by two-thirds (Goal 4 and 5) are also linked to some of the actions under the previous goals. However, the negative trends in these areas are also linked to the availability and accessibility of health services. The strategies to move forward include: establishing national policies, standards, and regulatory mechanisms for safe motherhood and developing systems to ensure their implementation; promoting appropriate community practices; monitoring maternal and newborn health care status and access to services; supporting programmes for immunization; the use of ORS, nutrition and water and sanitation interventions.

It took about forty years from 1960 to achieve a 50 percent reduction in child mortality. The MDG proposes a further two-thirds reduction by 2015, from ninety-three children of every 1,000 in 1990 dying before they were five to thirty-one of every 1,000 in 2015. However, recent articles in the *Lancet* show that the inter-regional variations are more startling, the gap between industrialized countries and sub-Saharan Africa being twenty-nine fold (6 and 175 respectively). In South Asia, one in every ten children dies before their fifth birthday. The task force for child mortality of the Millennium Project, considered the overall global picture worrisome with 10.8 million children under the age of five dying each year and mortality rates rising in some countries. The picture of maternal mortality is still more "worrisome." Overall levels of maternal mortality remains "stubbornly high," with approximately 530,000 deaths per year. One woman in every 16 may die of pregnancy-related complications as compared to one in every 2800 in developed countries. Such high differentials cannot be explained by availability of medical facilities alone and often larger social determinants are involved. Therefore, there is a need for a comprehensive approach which considers important social determinants of such high mortality rate under which issues related to health service components as well as medical interventions could be addressed (Nayar, 2007).

Parallel and disease-specific interventions which may emerge from the need to meet the MDGs or other goals could result in "duplications, distortions, disruptions and distractions" within the health care system (Travis et al., 2004). Another possibility is that selective approaches could be used as an excuse to give fillip to privatization even in extremely important areas like maternity care in rural areas. This is already proposed in India, where there is a move to involve private corporate sector in maternity care in rural areas in the name of reducing maternal mortality rate which could result in increasing the inequity in health care. Even in progressive states such as Kerala and in many other states as well, there are shifts towards a market-driven model and techno-managerial approaches such as Secondary Health Systems Project (Nayar and Nair, 2006). The redefinition of the state's role in healthcare as a regulatory and coordinating agency and not as a provider reveals that the neo-liberal visions have finally caught up with policy-makers of the so-called progressive state. Long-term, broader, system-based interventions through an integrated approach could be more cost-effective, result-oriented, and beneficial compared to such intensive drives especially in a context riddled with wider social disparities and inequities and to deal with emergence of new diseases and epidemiological patterns.

CONTEXTUALIZATION AND SOCIAL DISPARITIES

There is increasing evidence that strategies and organizational structures that work well in market economies may not be appropriate in low-income countries (Sen, 2003). Division of existing comprehensive approach into curative and preventive care and entrusting them with private and public sectors respectively, encouraging privatization or even a public-private mix, other forms of managerial practices intended for cost recovery etc., may in fact lead to negative fallouts in a society riddled with mass poverty and social inequalities including extreme stratification based on caste. The debates on reforms that have emerged in recent years are not just limited to the contextual differences which are certainly important as against a globalised vision, but even focus on the need to take into cognizance societal structures especially given the close linkages between social dimensions and health. There is already enough data to substantiate disparities between different social groups in India with regard to health. It appears that these disparities are persistent even in the post-reform era when claims are made about an all-around shining economy as indicated in tables 3.3, 3.4, and 3.5.

In the Indian context, caste may be considered as the most important indicator of social exclusion and broadly as a proxy for socio-economic status and poverty. In the identification of the poor, scheduled caste and scheduled tribes and in some cases the other backward castes are considered as socially disadvantaged groups and such groups have a higher probability of living under adverse conditions and poverty. The health status and utilization patterns of such groups give an indication of their social exclusion as well as an idea of the linkages between poverty and health. We examined broad linkages between caste and some select health/health utilization indicators. We examined data on infant mortality rate, utilization of maternal health care and childhood vaccinations among different caste groups in India. The data based on the National Family Health Survey highlight the caste differentials in health.

Table 3.3. Caste differentials with respect to IMR and Under 5 mortality in NFHS 1, 2, and 3

	Social Groups	*NFHS-1 (1992–93)*	*NFHS-2 (1998–99)*	*NFHS-3 (2005–06)*
Infant Mortality Rate	SC	107.3	83	71
	ST	90.5	84.2	63.9
	OBC	NA	76	61.1
	Others	82.2	61.8	55.7
Under 5 Mortality Rate	SC	149.1	119.3	94.7
	ST	135.2	126.6	99.8
	OBC	NA	103.1	78.7
	Others	111.5	82.6	68.2

Source: International Institute for Population Sciences and ORC Macro, 1995; 2000; 2007. NA: Not Available

There are considerable differences between different caste groups regarding infant mortality and under-five mortality. The difference between scheduled caste and the other castes (consisting of upper castes) stand out in the table in both the above variables (table 3.3).

Regarding accessibility variables, the other castes (the upper castes) are better-off in the case of maternity care. The proportion of scheduled caste and scheduled tribe women who have not availed any antenatal care is considerably higher compared to other castes. Utilization of doctors is also comparatively lower among these sections (table 3.4). Regarding childhood vaccinations, complete coverage is lowest among the scheduled castes followed by the scheduled tribes (table 3.5).

On the whole, the data suggest that the marginalized sections such as scheduled castes/scheduled tribes and the other backward castes who are also

Table 3.4. Percentage of utilization of antenatal care by social groups in India

Sources of antenatal care	*Social groups*	*NFHS-1 (1992–93)*	*NFSH-2 (1998–99)*	*NFSH-3 (2005–06)*
ANC at home from health workers	SC	14.6	5.9	NA
	ST	18.5	10.0	NA
	OBC	NA	5.9	NA
	Others	11.9	4.0	NA
Doctors	SC	29.4	41.7	42.0
	ST	21.0	34.7	32.8
	OBC	NA	48.9	48.4
	Others	44.0	56.5	63.6
Other health professionals	SC	12.8	13.3	0.7
	ST	7.1	11.5	1.0
	OBC	NA	9.6	0.8
	Others	9.1	10.6	1.6
Traditional birth attendants and others	SC	0.2	0.2	1.5
	ST	0.2	0.3	2.3
	OBC	NA	0.2	0.7
	Others	0.3	0.2	1.1
No ANC	SC	42.2	38.2	25.9
	ST	52.3	43.1	29.4
	OBC	NA	34.8	25.5
	Others	34.0	27.9	15.2

Source: International Institute for Population Sciences and ORC Macro, 1995; 2000; 2007 NA: Not Available

Table 3.5. Percentage of childhood vaccination coverage by social groups in India

Vaccination	*Social Groups*	*NFHS-1 (1992–93)*	*NFHS -2 (1998–99)*	*NFHS-3 (2005–06)*
BCG	SC	52.9	69.6	75.4
	ST	50.2	60.0	71.7
	OBC	NA	71.6	76.4
	Others	65.2	76.1	84.1
Polio 0 dose	SC	3.5	11.7	46.8
	ST	2.7	4.5	30.9
	OBC	NA	18.7	46.2
	Others	5.0	11.6	57.6
DPT 1	SC	58.7	68.4	74.2
	ST	52.9	57.0	65.9
	OBC	NA	72.4	74.1
	Others	69.2	76.4	82.6
DPT 2	SC	51.4	52.7	64.6
	ST	45.4	37.5	53.2
	OBC	NA	56.7	63.9
	Others	62.2	60.4	75.8
DPT 3	SC	43.3	82.6	51.9
	ST	36.5	73.9	40.9
	OBS	NA	86.6	52.6
	Others	55.0	84.6	65.4
Polio 1	SC	60.2	77.8	92.2
	ST	54.7	66.9	86.8
	OBC	NA	81.3	94.4
	Others	69.6	79.4	94.0
Polio 2	SC	53.0	61.3	88.6
	ST	47.6	49.0	79.8
	OBC	NA	65.6	90.3
	Others	64.2	65.6	89.7
Polio 3	SC	44.4	47.6	76.3
	ST	37.6	34.3	64.6
	OBC	NA	50.7	81.4
	Others	56.8	57.1	79.6
Measles	SC	33.9	40.2	56.7
	ST	32.7	24.2	46.1
	OBC	NA	11.6	55.4
	Others	44.7	13.3	68.8
All	SC	26.8	15.1	39.7
	ST	24.8	24.5	31.3
	OBC	NA	33.4	40.7
	Others	38.2	38.1	53.8

Source: International Institute for Population Sciences and ORC Macro, 1995; 2000; 2007 NA: Not Available

the poor in India suffer from a "social gap" (and not just a wealth gap alone) in terms of health status and health services. It can be broadly observed based on the available data that the reforms and targeting have not benefited these marginalized sections.

THE NEW FORMS OF NEO-LIBERAL REFORMS

As against managerial reforms and disinvestment, Indian health services are also witnessing new forms of financing models such as micro-insurance and community-based insurance. These new ways of mainly financing are suggested to address the increasing non-availability, non-accessibility, and non-affordability of health services. These are old medicines in new bottles and as discussed in chapter 2, the Indian state was already predisposed to such changes as such preferences existed even among the members of the Bhore committee. The ruling classes in India and the increasing numbers of middle classes were also ideologically predisposed to the content of these reforms.

The Coming of the Insurance Model

It is often assumed uncritically that the private sector is more efficient than the public sector health services. This myth has now been admitted by a recent World Bank document at least with respect to insurance which states that the private insurance costs are extremely high compared to public insurance given the high marketing costs. Similarly, in Singapore, it has been shown that private hospitals charge much more high charges for services of comparable quality as those provided by the public hospitals (Hsiao and Heller, 2007).

In recent years, advocacy regarding the need to adopt an insurance model in health care is becoming strong despite lack of adequate evidence of its applicability in low-income countries (Preker et. al, 2002). In the Indian case, the out-of-pocket expenditure by households is pointed out as a reason for introducing risk-pooling strategies. However, data given in table 3.6 shows that the private sector expends only 5.73 percent of funds for health care as against nearly 20 percent by the state. Logically therefore, it can be argued that the high out-of-pocket expenses by households is due to low investment by the state. The same data is also used as a rationale for privatization by arguing that the people are already spending money from their pockets and therefore it is a profitable sector.

Community based health insurance has been proposed as a transitional mechanism to achieving universal coverage for health care in low-income

Table 3.6. Source of funds and proportion of expenditure for health care in India 2004-5

Sector	*%Expenditure*
Central	6.78%
State	11.97%
Local bodies	0.92%
Households	71.13%
Private firms	5.73%
NGOs	0.07%
External support	2.28%

Source: Government of India, 2009b

countries on the basis of policy link between CBHI and universal coverage established by the historical experience of mutual health insurance in countries such as Germany and Japan in the 19th century (Mladovsky and Mossialos, 2006). The CBHI may be different from the three models that exist at present such as: direct reimbursement model-post-hoc payment of money as in France-Switzerland; contract models—the company contracts providers for the clients as in Germany and; integrated models—the insurer provides the service to the insured as in British NHS (government) and US HMO (private). The missing link in the present models of insurance including CBHI is the entirely different social context. Context-dependent policy considerations such as values of scheme members and people in their communities, community goals and local and regional power relations are not emphasized in the analysis of CBHI by institutions such as the World Bank and the WHO (Mladovsky and Mossialos, 2006).

There are also suggestions to implement pro-poor micro insurance schemes in India and evidence base regarding this approach is being generated (ECCP project, 2005). Micro health insurance is basically a financing scheme that has three key features: community control, voluntary membership, and prepayment for health care by community members (Hsiao 2004). The essential feature is that it is small in size and in the extent of contribution and coverage. Although basically intended for the poor in overcoming the resource crunch of families at the time illness, the market for health care is the basic principle on which some of the recommendations are made. For instance, the proposal on pro-poor insurance scheme is based on the financial logic that more than half of the people at the bottom of the pyramid spend more than Rs. 2400 per annum. In aggregate terms this is a huge figure and offers a "sustainable business" for insurance companies (Update, 2005). Another argument in favor of micro health insurance (MHI) is the impact in terms of impoverishment of households due to healthcare costs which has been also termed as catastrophic health expenditure. It is generally accepted now that out of pocket expenditure can adversely affect overall socio-economic conditions of the poor especially when it is a catastrophic expenditure for an illness. Most advocacies regarding introduction of private care or insurance model is based on this logic that poor people already spend money for buying health care. In a recent study by the Kerala Sastra Sahitya Parishad (KSSP), it was found that families below the poverty line spend more than one third of their income for treatment. This is substantial as against 10 percent by the families belonging to the upper middle class. The study also shows that although morbidity load is declining, the per capita expenditure is steeply rising. It is generally assumed that a community based micro insurance scheme will be able to tackle the pauperization due to catastrophic health expenditure (KSSP, 2006).

However, some of the constraints identified for the micro health insurance are: prohibitive level of surplus requirement, inability of micro schemes to transfer risks to reinsurance, lack of information, almost no support in raising technical and administrative skills at micro insurance level (and the funds to finance training), and complications in ensuring ample supply of medical services of good quality at affordable cost. There are also regulations which force these micro-health insurance institutions to be mere agents of commercial insurance companies (ECCP project, 2005). The four-pronged strategy suggested to overcome these barriers are: (i) Flexible benefit package design, reflecting local priorities and ability to pay; (ii) Reinsurance of micro health insurance units; (iii) Subsidies to cover part of the cost of the insurance premium and/or the reinsurance premium; and (iv) capacity building at micro insurance level (ECCP project, 2005). In India, 8 million individuals were covered under micro health insurance in about twenty schemes in states such as Karnataka, Tamil Nadu, Gujarat, Chattisgarh, Maharastra, and West Bengal.

Various insurance packages were initiated by the central and state governments such as Kerala. The *Kudumbu Suraksha* program of the government of Kerala was to be implemented by the ICICI Lombard, a commercial insurance company. The high morbidity rate and the prevalence of diseases such as leptospirosis, dengue, gastro-intestinal diseases apart from other poverty and water-related diseases and their impact on the economic conditions of the poor are pointed out as reasons for initiating an insurance scheme for the poor in Kerala. The identification criteria used for the *kudumbhasree* program (which is an income generating self-help program; see chapter 5) was proposed to be used for the above program as well. However, this did not take off in its original format.

The Rashtriya Swasthya Bima Yojana (RSBY) is one of the state-led micro-insurance health schemes in India which was evolved in 2008 under the Ministry of Labour and Employment based on the earlier experiences mainly to guard people belonging to below poverty line (BPL) from illness shocks (Swarup and Jain, 2012). The beneficiaries are covered for hospitalization expenses up to Rs. 30,000. The main objectives of the RSBY are to:

- provide financial security to below poverty line families which is expected to be 300 million for hospitalization related expenses
- improve access to quality health care
- provide beneficiaries the power of choice to select a health care provider
- provide a scheme which is simple to use for the beneficiaries and which transparent

As against private insurance, pre-existing conditions are fully covered and there is no age limit. The beneficiaries pay a registration fee of Rs.30 and the premiums are paid by the central (75 percent) and state governments (25 percent) to the insurer selected by competitive bidding. The RSBY also works on the same governance model as HIV/AIDS or many components of the NRHM where an independent nodal agency (a para-state organization) is set up to oversee the implementation and on a public-private partnership model. Although, the RSBY experience is under a concurrent evaluation, some broad trends could be obtained. The major problem is with the BPL categorization, large scale exclusion and inclusion errors and issue of BPL cards which led to major resentments at the village levels which also reduced enrollment (Palacios, 2010). Other issues include problems universally associated with insurance such as moral hazards and sudden increase in hospitalization (which is assumed to be due to repressed demands). The male-female differentials are also pointed out but in the second year, the male bias has reduced to a large extent. Predictably, the increase in demand is to be met by empanelling more private hospitals. Some of the challenges pointed out in evaluation studies and overviews are 1) increased provider induced demands; 2) sub-optimal provider payment systems; 3) problems due to hospital accreditation and quality control, etc. (Palacios, 2010). There are also complaints about lack of compliance and frauds committed by private hospitals. Narayana analyzed the enrollment of the poor under RSBY in its third year of operation and concluded that the possibility of covering all the poor by 2012 appeared unlikely. He pointed out that it is difficult to assess the average increase in hospitalization rates due to exceptionally high rates in a few districts (Narayana, 2010). The high rates could be due to the facility to access private hospitals under RSBY. Due to non-availability and absence of such facilities in other districts, this may not be achieved in other districts. It has been also observed that insurance companies do some skimming by enrolling only one member of the household as the companies get payment on household basis and not individual basis (Das and Leino, 2011). There is also no information on the interphase between those enrolled and the hospitals including the pattern of treatment they received. There was no way to ascertain whether hospitalization was necessary. There are cases in which members were advised hospitalization on paper as the benefits are not given for outpatient services in some states.

Critiques point out that such models only help in facilitating unregulated commercialization of health care and commodification of the body (Prasad and Raghavendra, 2012). The neo-liberal insurance model of health care such as the Aarogyasri in the state of Andhra Pradesh which inspired such an approach in many other states of India has only helped in further weakening the public health sector and strengthening the private and corporate sectors. It appears that the insurance model has now been taken over by the neo-liberal advocates of universal health care (UHC) as well. The three "I's": Investment, Institutional reforms, and Insurance are the latest mantra for achieving universal health care for them. Needless to say that such an approach to universalize health care will only lead to further disorder in health services and therefore, an alternative approach to UHC is needed.

Public-Private Partnerships (PPP)

The move toward public-private partnerships (PPP) was initiated primarily on the assumption of inefficiency of the state but it tries to flag the advantages of both the sectors. The assumption is that the public sector has the network, manpower and a social obligation while the private sector has efficiency, transparency, technology, and resources to deliver. The primacy of profits for the private sector is not highlighted here. The model is purely based on a deduction that the PPP is combining the good of two sectors to achieve an objective ignoring the evils which are much more annihilating as far as private sector is considered. Policy implications are drawn from insufficient evidence regarding utilization of private sector for delivering core public health programs such as tuberculosis control (Montagu et al., 2011). It is suggested that legal and fiscal support be given to private facilities and contracting out services to the private sector be explored as a viable alternative to the public sector. Such prescriptive studies which implicitly support neo-liberal mechanisms are fortunately declining.

Similar to the insurance model, reviews and reports have pointed out several problems in evolving such models which suggest contracting out to the private sector or partnership with them for delivering essential health services such as maternity care. A draft report of a task group for PPP under NRHM points out the need for a credible public system, strict regulation and control, and to distinguish not for profit and for profit non-governmental sector (Government of India, 2006b). The report notes that there is no short cut to a well-funded, well-functioning, efficient, and effective public sector in health care from the sub-center to the district level. The task group also points out that the health improvement witnessed in states such as Kerala, Tamil Nadu, Himachal Pradesh, etc. can be largely attributed to the public sector and therefore what is required is a re-crafting of the public sector to increase efficiency, accountability, and decentralized governance.

The evidence regarding the availability, accessibility, and quality of the private sector to people who are impoverished should be the starting point for public-private partnerships. Especially, when it comes to health, the most important issue is the social function of the state which may not fit into private sector interests and therefore a partnership with such a sector will not lead to optimization of the social function and will dilute the obligation of the state to its people.

Indian Public Health Standard (IPHS)

It is a set of measures to improve quality of health services at various levels such as sub-centre, primary health center, community health center, sub-district and sub-divisional hospitals, and the district hospitals. The main agenda under the revised guidelines issued in 2012 is to ensure quality assurance which is a new reform induced program and is largely curative oriented. The guidelines have been categorized according to the services offered at various levels which consider minimum assured services which should be in place and a set of projected services. In the case of sub centers, the IPHS identifies two types: Type A where institutional deliveries will not be available and Type B where such facilities are available apart from all preventive, promotive, and some curative services. A model citizen's charter and constitution of Village Health Sanitation and Nutrition Committee with involvement of Panchati Raj institutions are also part of the IPH standard (Government of India, 2012a). The case load of deliveries constitute the basis of categorizing primary health centers (PHC) into type A (less than 20 deliveries in a month) and type B (more than twenty deliveries in a month). The projected standard for PHCs is forty patients per doctor per day and about 60 percent utilization of the six beds and the fulfillment of the expected number for maternal and child health and family planning. Rogi Kalyan Samiti/Primary Health Centre Management Committee has also been included as the standard. Minimum standards in terms of availability of instruments, medicines, and services for each of the national programs for disease control have also been evolved (Government of India, 2012b). Community health centers have been considered as gatekeepers of referral services in the district. In addition to already prescribed specialists such as surgery, medicine, obstetrics, and gynecology, and pediatrics, the guidelines suggest inclusion of anesthetist and a public health specialist (Government of India, 2012c). A block public health unit with a block medical officer, a public health specialist and a public health nurse has been included in the new standard.

For sub-divisional hospitals and district hospitals, the standards are more curative oriented and based on the case load of the institution. The main focus is on newborn care, specialty services such as psychiatry, physical medicine and rehabilitation, accident and trauma services, integrated counseling and testing center, and post natal services. The guidelines include the pattern for hospital building, planning and layout, display of signage, disaster prevention measures for new facilities, barrier free access, and environmental friendly features. The guidelines also suggest rationalization of existing manpower and new manpower for physical medicine and rehabilitation services, dental, and immunization services. Apart from these, national guidelines on hospital waste management, Guidelines to reduce environmental pollution due to mercury waste, and Seismic safety guidelines have been included (Government of India 2012d). For district hospitals, in addition to some of the above standards, surgical procedures, super specialties, and diagnostic facilities are also included especially in those with more than 300 beds. The minimum assured services include those related to OPD, indoor and emergency services. Dialyses services and anti-retro viral treatments are the projected services for the district hospitals (Government of India, 2012e).

The IPHS is a desirable standard for achieving the minimum essential services in the health services especially at the peripheral levels. However, given the current manpower situation in the country especially for support staff and specialist doctors, these could be difficult propositions and are unlikely to be achieved in the near future.

Conceptual Shifts in Public Health Practice

One of the important implications of the organizational reforms discussed in the previous sections is the concomitant shifts that they have induced in public health concepts and practice in the country. The opening up of medical care to the private sector and public hospitals to private investment led to commercialization of medical care thereby underplaying the role of social sector and welfare strategies (Qadeer and Nayar, 2005). As a result, "the

WHO started changing the theoretical basis of public health itself. Thus instead of the state's responsibility the emphasis shifted on public-private partnerships. No more the environment (physical, social, and economic) was the key concern. Attention was shifted to individual responsibility and behavior rather than crucial social dimensions. The broader integrated approach of the past was replaced by the purely technology based interventions and that too for diseases for which the MNCs had something to offer. Primary health care approach based on affordability, needs, and self-sufficiency was rejected by the slogan of interdependence of a globalized world. The use of DALYS that erased the difference between death and life and separated diseases into isolated entities was used to change the image of disease patterns. Putting non-communicable diseases high up in the priority list, it served to increase profits as it enriches the pharmaceutical companies and diagnostic industry (Ibid.:66-67). These conceptual changes are very often uncritically accepted which not only influence health care but also influence medical education and shaping of future doctors.

Qadeer argues that in the present dispensation leading to penetration of international capital directly to sub-regions, states are losing their autonomy and increasingly they are being considered as clients of aid and loan market (Qadeer, 2005). In this process, they are also turned into mere stewards and not as guardians of welfare for their citizens. All these have serious implications for the delivery of health services and family planning as well as for medical research and education.

The changing role of the state also means new strategies in the entire levels of public health in terms of curative, preventive, promotive, and rehabilitative services. New essential packaging of care for cost-cutting and prioritization of problems suiting pharmaceutical corporations and international funding agencies are trends which influence the strategies. The apparently receding state also means new micro-strategies such as shifting the focus from population which is the conventional domain of public health to the family and the individual. Such shifting focus is in tune with the insurance models being advocated now.

The emphasis of health programs is on prevention of easily preventable diseases through techno-centric interventions such as the pulse polio program. The one approach being implicitly advised is the categorical approach where problems are taken-up one by one rather than handled in a comprehensive way. Over reliance on technology and such selective handling of diseases mean marginalization of poverty-health linkage in public health discourse.

One of the most critiqued is the shifts in strategy from primary health care (PHC) to a packaged selective care (Qadeer, 2001). The PHC is based on a framework which ensures equity in health care about participation of the people in socially acceptable services. It also reiterates state responsibility for delivering affordable technologies in basic, secondary, and tertiary care. The packaged selective care is rooted in a different notion of public health driven by the market and takes public health to the biomedical model. For instance, the new language of health economics such as risk-pooling etc., has dominated public health discourse in the post-nineties. Many of the reform packages discussed in this chapter also fall under such a framework.

Another major conceptual change is the emergence of evidence-based medicine (EBM). This is normally suggested by the advocates who are interested in pushing technical solutions and proximal or downstream factors rather than the more difficult distal or upstream factors. The criticisms are also directed at the unbridled objectivism and scientism in evidence-based medicine (Mykhalovskiy and Weir, 2004). From a political economy tradition, EBM is critiqued as a mechanism which serves the interest of the capital as it ignores the larger social and environmental factors while focusing on the individual patient. Some scholars think that these are dangerous innovations which are used to usher in cost-cutting mechanisms (Sackett et al., 1996). Although its emergence was in relation to clinical medicine, the approach was applied to public health practices, approaches, and programs. This meant that any strategy has to be adopted only on the basis of evidence regarding its effectiveness and efficiency which can be measured. "It is now widely accepted that much of the 'scientific' evidence in health care is of extremely poor quality, biased in favor of professional or commercial sponsors, producing misleading and unreliable results that overstate the benefits and play down the harms of many health care interventions" (Moynihan, 2004:3). According to Moynihan, evidence could be categorized based on the way it is used such as instrumental—where relevant research results are used for policy decision-making; selective or instrumental—where evidence is used to justify or sustain a pre-determined decision; and finally, the enlightening—which helps in enriching the understanding of a problem. The selective care (or selective PHC as it is known) packages or as mentioned earlier, many packages which were implemented as a part of health reforms fall into the second category. Apart from EBM, there is also eminence based medicine which is doctor-centric or technically driven. The current corporate medicine is largely eminence based which includes decision-making based on not just the doctors but even those dependent on machines and technology.

Despite the hype and rhetoric of EBM, what becomes primary is politics which decides what kind of evidence is produced, heard, or used (Bambra, 2013). It is now realized that pure evidence is impossible to be translated into policy given the political imperatives and the complexities involved in policy-making. Probably, this marks the end of simplistic, linear, and technocratic-driven public health policy-making.

The policy making context even in health care which involves a larger technical dimension is political and a number of actors, factors, and forces influence such decisions (Bowen and Zwi, 2005). It is also important to understand the role of values in areas such as health inequities where actions are not taken despite availability of strong evidence. Similarly, preference for certain technologies including reproductive technologies despite clear evidence regarding their side effects is again a political and ideological issue.

As already mentioned in this section, there is a renewed focus on individuals and their behavior in recent policies and strategies with respect to general well-being as well as in disease control programs. It starts with the notions of creating happiness and life satisfaction although it is known that rising incomes do not correlate with happiness as evident from the US where GNP per capita has risen three-fold from the sixties but the measures of happiness have not changed (Helliwell, Layard, and Sachs, 2012). After having created crises and turmoil, now the neo-liberal palliative is to create synthetic happiness using individual approaches. In this happiness project, the interest to create happiness in a gloomy world riddled by crises and turmoil appears to be justified as a humanitarian agenda. In fact, even the international philanthropic organizations have shown a keen interest in defining the notions and approaches which facilitate happiness so that apparently the sadness can be wiped off.

In health, the individual approaches have a great following and a long history. The family planning program consolidated and reinforced the individual-centered as against population-centered approaches which was the easiest way to blame the victim. This was by evolving health/extension education and behavior modification programs.

The behavioral approaches that evolved out of its predecessors such as health education was tried tested misused or overused in different contexts. Such a strategy has also been part of the academic or non-academic developmental approaches. But the most dominant feature of this approach was its paternalistic outlook, an outlook that focuses on provision of services—to be handed over to the users by knowledgeable and technically "superior" people. This outlook also assumes that failure of people to appropriate the services means lack of knowledge, awareness or education. Such an approach therefore has a number of technical paraphernalia to make people aware of the "goodness" of the services handed over to them with different names such as extension education, health education, IEC approach, behavior change communication, etc. The behavior change communication (BCC) also gained ground due to the sudden outbreak of HIV/AIDS in pandemic proportions but it was extended to nutrition, sanitation, immunization, etc. The root cause of this was located in the risky behavior of individuals which then became the main strategy of HIV/AIDS control programs.

The HIV/AIDS program gave legitimacy to behavior change as it assumed that the risk behavior is the main culprit for the disease. According to behavior theorists, targeting specific behaviors such as "walking for twenty minutes a day" will be more effective than general behavioral categories (exercise) or goals (weight reduction). In HIV/AIDS, the focus thus shifted to use of condoms for sex to use of condoms for specific acts of sex such as "using a condom for vaginal sex with one's spouse or main partner is a very different behavior to always using a condom for vaginal sex with a commercial sex worker, or always using a condom for anal sex with one's spouse" (Fishbein, 2000:273-274). According to Fishbein, there are four elements in any given behavior: the action (use of condom), the target (actual use of condom), the context (anal sex with regular partner or vaginal sex with a commercial sex worker), and the time period in which the behavior is expected to occur (always or irregular use). Other key questions regarding the suitability of behavior change communication are: 1) It is difficult to translate the effectiveness seen in small group clinical trials into the real world effectiveness as most of the clinical trials have occurred in high-income countries using intensive, professional program models which may not apply to resource poor settings. 2) The generalizability of even evidence from the real world settings cannot be transferred to other communities, sub-groups, and types of epidemics. 3) Even sustaining behavior change over longer periods is also difficult as it is found that the favorable change can fade away over time. In many countries, it was difficult to preserve the prevention climate when the disease become less threatening. 4) Most of the models of behavior change are based on cognitive behavioral theories which assume that individuals will take steps to avoid risks. However, it is also evident that most of the behaviors are heavily influenced by environmental, cultural and social factors. The behavioral interventions are not been sufficiently informed by social and ethnographic research. 5) Most of the interventions are based on discrete variables without acknowledging the comprehensiveness of control strategies (Global HIV prevention working group, 2008). In existing behavior change models, these complexities are not recognized and therefore they exist as vertical interventions and often reduce itself to rituals.

Uttar Pradesh is one of the first states in India to initiate a BCC strategy under the National Rural Health Mission (Government of Uttar Pradesh, 2008: 10). This involved an exercise which started with defining the behavioral actions that required to be addressed in the strategy followed by assessing the barriers which exist in the state for change. The strategy also tried to address the issue of making health services available and accessible to the marginalized communities. The strategy also tried use persuasive techniques to integrate new practices into the existing social environment.

The UP strategy is a curious mix of the ancient Indian theory of communication known as *sadharanikaran* with the John Hopkins University sponsored *pathways* model. "*Sadharanikaran* means simplification without dilution; simplification while maintaining the essence and meaning of the content that is to be communicated. It is among the few theories of behavior and communication that has its origins outside of Anglo-American culture, thereby providing a perspective quite different from the 'cognitive-rationally' driven theories that predominate the field" (Ibid.:11). The UP strategy on BCC has the following priority areas selected after a situation analysis. Apart from these stated priorities, the introduction section in the document reveals that family planning including female sterilization and IUD insertions dominates the target of BCC approach. Evidence shows that many of these variables have a larger social component than behavioral and therefore such strategies may not work unless an integrated approach is not implemented.

1. Antenatal care
2. Institutional deliveries
3. Post natal & newborn care
4. Married adolescents
5. Gender discrimination (female foeticide, infant girl, under 5 girl, son preference and therefore large family size)
6. Unmet need for family planning
7. Nutrition through the life cycle (infant, under three, adolescent, woman)
8. Routine immunization
9. Hygiene and safe water practices
10. Marginalized groups and households including urban poor
11. Need for supportive supervision of Accredited Social Health Activists (ASHA)
12. Capacity building of BCC skills for service providers across National Rural Health Mission
13. Workload definition and structuring of workload for the ASHAs

The individual orientation has also gained ground in recent times due to the so-called epidemiological shifts to non-communicable diseases where the causative factors are located in the life style of people. This has a great market potential as well where exercises and healthy foods are commoditized. This was also used to market exercise machines and weight reduction techniques. All these approaches also focus on individual psyche in some way as the dimension to alter and to be made amenable, approachable and accessible to the programs designed by the superior minds. The "synthetic" character of such needs is quite evident.

Another evolving concept is known as global health which advocates universal strategies for grappling with public health problems. The Stockholm declaration for global health urges countries and the institutions to act in several areas within the post-MDG context from 2015. Basically, there are four areas in which the global health agenda wants to focus on (Friberg et al., 2012:2066):

> *Linking ongoing agendas with new agendas*
> Ensure that the post-2015 development agenda builds on current MDGs, is universal and incorporates emerging challenges. These include socioeconomic and gender inequalities, non-communicable diseases (such as heart disease, stroke, diabetes, cancer, and chronic respiratory disease), and climate change (including threats to food and water security).
>
> *Creating stronger leadership and accountability so that health is at the center of development*
> Ensure that health is a high-profile unifying theme in the post-2015 development agenda, positioned to act as a catalyst for human rights and global solidarity; and that appropriate accountability mechanisms and professional leadership for global and national commitments are established.
>
> *Building capacity and investing in health*
> Invest in leadership for global health through education from primary school to university, and enable public empowerment by bringing together networks for intersectoral multidisciplinary research and action on global health.
>
> *Exploiting opportunities and synergies*
> Identify and exploit opportunities for applying effective democratic principles to ongoing health agendas (including maternal, child, and mental health), violence, climate change, and other emerging challenges, thus bringing sustainable social, ecological, and economic short-term and long-term returns for both public and private sectors. Pursue synergies such as health and climate cobenefits that bring multiple gains.

Unfortunately, the global health process is dominated by the Western institutions, think tanks, expert groups, and high-level meetings which could result in global thinking being imposed on local levels (Friberg et al., 2012). This could end up similar to the earlier calls such as "think globally, act locally" where international experts and donors think and local functionaries act!

EVOLVING SCENARIOS

Against this backdrop of individual-centric strategies and decontextualized global strategies, there are positive signals as well in the renewed focus on social determinants. The role of social and economic dimensions in health improvement is now axiomatic despite problems in evolving a universal probabilistic framework due to the influence of several contextual variables. Empirical examinations of the linkages between socio-economic factors such as poverty, income, occupation, class, etc. have a long history (Krieger, 2005). Chadwick's pioneering work on the sanitary condition of laboring population in Great Britain indicated that non-biomedical factors are responsible for the occurrence of disease and pestilence in the 19th century. McKeown's convincing thesis on the role of non-biomedical determinants for the decline of mortality rates in England and Wales during the 19th century reinforced these linkages which led to further examination of the linkages between environment, socio-economic changes, and disease trends (McKeown, 1976). The search for environmental and social determinants of disease was not fashionable topic and carried little scientific prestige at one point in time (Dubos, 1965). As Dubos remarked, "history alone need not provide the evidence of disease patterns differing and changing rapidly with environmental and social conditions. A spectacular proof of this relationship emerges from a comparison of mortality and morbidity rates, as well as type of diseases, recorded in our own times for different countries and different social groups" (Dubos, 1968). Despite early reservations, considerable research evidence has further reinforced these linkages. Michael Marmot argues that the environment shaped by social and economic organization is partly responsible for the status of health and factors such as ill-health and childhood environment, the work environment, unemployment, patterns of social relationships, social exclusion, food, addictive behavior, transport, etc. do account for the differences in disease rates within and between countries (Marmot, 1999). They also create problems for the medical care system. The equality question came into prominence when Richard Wilkinson proposed the relative income hypothesis, maintaining that societies with wider income differences show lower levels of average health than societies with greater income equality (Wilkinson, 1996). An approach to social determinants is therefore, not rhetorical but has to be part of a wider strategy to grapple with the problem of ill-health.

Poverty and health linkages need to be understood with a broader social determinants framework. The interest in understanding social determinants was revived after the 1986 Ottawa Charter of Health Promotions which recognized peace, shelter, education, food, income, a harmonious eco-system, resources, social justice and equity as essential pre-requisites for health (WHO, 1986). Despite such a forceful international charter, the approach to social determinants remained extremely individualized and behavioral.

A structural orientation was missing in policy prescriptions in developing and developed countries (Raphael, 2006). Considerable background and conceptual work have been completed and the final report of the commission is now available and a series of follow-up actions have been already undertaken. It is now well-accepted that poverty, quality of life, employment, working, and living conditions influence health. It means that behavioral modifications and health education will have a limited impact on improving health status unless the larger structural issues which sustain inequality are addressed. The current interest in poverty and health stems from this recognition.

The linkages between poverty and health have also become important after the declaration of the Millennium Development Goals (MDGs) by the United Nations discussed earlier in this chapter. According to the MDG goal on poverty, the member countries are expected to halve the proportion of people living on less than a dollar a day and those who suffer from hunger. Strategies for moving forward include: support for country-led economic and social initiatives that focus on poverty reduction; strengthening capabilities to provide basic social services; and assisting capacity building for assessment, monitoring, and planning. The basic approach does not involve any re-orientation or restructuring of the economic policies. It is based on poverty reduction strategies mainly involving instrumentalist programs such as school meal schemes, take-home rations, and supplementary feeding programs which are considered to be cross-cutting, solutions. Alleviation of hunger is also another objective under this with the objective of increasing labor productivity and earning capacity of individuals. Many critiques feel that it is unrealistic to achieve considerable reduction in the proportion of poor without focusing on a viable distributive policy on food and land. One cannot expect to improve access to nutritionally adequate food for the poor through agricultural production, agricultural trade, and the overall trade policies alone (Nayar and Razum, 2006).

Need for a Contextual Approach in Social Determinants

The social determinants need to be contextualized with regard to individual countries of the region. This is the most crucial, challenging and complex task as there are many specific factors for which actions have to be undertaken within countries and regions within countries. A distinction may be made between countries where there considerable decline in the indicators in line with the MDG 4 and 5 has been observed and those countries where the rates are worrisome such as India, Pakistan, Bangladesh, Myanmar, Bhutan, etc. It is evident that in the latter countries, an action program with an appropriate balance between biomedical and social dimensions may be evolved. The social, cultural, behavioral, institutional, and technological factors should form the pillars of such a contextual approach.

Gender

Gender is one of the important social dimensions which require a multidimensional approach especially considering maternal, neonatal, and child health (MNCH). The status of a woman in the society influences the decisions regarding a host of factors concerning her directly; the autonomy regarding marriage, sexuality and reproduction, contraception, and even decisions regarding health and health behavior. The differential treatment of males and females with regard to food and medical care and the discrimination that they face during early childhood have disastrous consequences for *MNCH. This has been repeatedly pointed out by many international publications* (World Bank, 1993). In recent years, this has been brought into the inequality agenda which essentially calls for specific interventions at the social sector which help in reducing the socio-economic inequalities. There are considerable evidence that gender inequity marked by differential access to resources, assets, and opportunities directly affects the welfare of women and children which work as an "archetypical inequality trap" for the women (World Bank, 2006).

The data on under 5 mortality rates for boys and girls for selected countries show that it is only in India that the female children have a higher mortality rate compared to boys (WHO, 2007). This calls for a closer look at the factors which may include unequal norms, and aspects of social structures including patriarchy preserved by marriage, inheritance, and kinship patterns. Obviously, inequality at home needs to be addressed very carefully by appropriate social policies. Contextual factors such as preference for male children are rooted in such patriarchal social structures which also result in adverse sex ratios in several north Indian states. Empowering the women by appropriate economic and social programs could be one of the ways to grapple with this "inequality trap" that the women face which may indirectly impact on health outcomes. However, such programs have to be more holistic than the ones which are implemented now focusing on income generation or economic activities.

Income Differentials and Socio-economic Status

Evidently, the most significant factor which has been emphasized repeatedly is the income inequality within countries (World Bank, 2006). Recent studies show striking association between socio-economic status of families and under 5 mortality rates in a population of children in 43 resource-poor countries. It is also found that the socio-economic inequality in child mortality is increasing in these countries (Irwin, Siddiqi, and Hertzman, 2007). Data from the four South Asian countries such as India, Pakistan, Bangladesh and Nepal show considerable gap between the highest wealth quintile and the lowest wealth quintile regarding under 5 child mortality (WHO, 2007). Again, the gap is more in India compared to the other countries.

There is enough evidence that behavioral practices including health actions are rooted in the social, political, and cultural context (Djurfeldt and Lindberg, 1976; Banerji, 1982; Basu, 1992). However, the specific pathways of such social variables and health are not well-researched which often results in half-baked and uni-focused actions such as behavioral change programs or educational activities. What is required is a more multi-focused action on vulnerable sections of the population which can not only take care of the specific social vulnerabilities such as unemployment, social exclusion, etc. but can also enhance accessibility and availability of health services.

Focus on Social Exclusion

It is quite evident that issues of gender, income differentials, religion/caste, etc. impinge on health status and contribute to poor MNCH outcomes. All these variables create conditions leading to social exclusion of large sections in the population. Economic capability (poverty), gender, age, caste and religion, education, etc. are important variables which indicate exclusion from social and economic opportunities. Social exclusion mainly refers to the inability of our society to keep all groups and individuals within reach of what we expect as society to realize their full potential. Marginalization of certain groups or classes occurs in most societies including developed countries and perhaps it is more pronounced in underdeveloped countries. DHS surveys in some countries of the region also show considerable difference between mothers who are illiterate and those with higher education with regard to under 5 mortality. However, this could be also due to the socio-economic differences between the two groups. Amartya Sen has pointed out that the concept of social exclusion has to also take into cognizance the issues regarding poverty and deprivation (Sen, 1999). From a policy perspective, considering the health inequality and social inequality inter-phase, the focus has to be on the poorer classes who have a higher risk for diseases as well as higher probability from being excluded from the health services. This is essential given the higher proportion of the poor as well as socially disadvantaged, the magnitude of health problems and the epidemiological profile in the society.

Health in All Policies (HiAP) and Intersectoral Approach

A number of regional factors—although linked to universal trends—are elucidated in a WHO study "Intersectoral linkages and health development" published in 1984 when some of the initiatives in the social sector undertaken in the previous decades had started showing results with regard to health status including indicators such as IMR, MMR, etc. (Gunatilleke, 1984). This was also the period when regional differences in health status in South-East Asia became prominent. The study clearly showed that actions taken in the social and economic sectors had considerable impacts on the state of health in the countries of the region.

The three cases in the region—Kerala state in India, Sri Lanka, and Thailand, which may be considered as success stories with regard to achieving better health status highlight the role of social dimensions and other intersectoral variables (See box No. 3.1, 3.2, and 3.3). It is evident that Sri Lanka and the Kerala state of India have considerable similarities where better health status was achieved by a redistribution policy as well as considerable inputs into activities which provided better living conditions for the poor and the marginalized. The case of Thailand and many other East Asian countries highlight the fact that growth-oriented development if sustained and followed-up with a basic need orientation could impact on the health status of the population. It is this diversity within the region which calls for a contextual approach. The need for understanding such diversities is also reinforced in a recent case study of 18 countries (WHO and PHAC, 2008).

TEXTBOX 3.1. INTERSECTORAL LINKAGES IN KERALA

- Redistribution policies in land which benefit poor peasants
- Effective public distribution system (PDS) which make available food, grains, and other essential items to the poor at a cheaper rate
- A selective program on housing which benefited landless labor
- Expanding a protected water supply program
- Higher investments in education

Source: Godfrey Gunatilleke (1984) Ed. Intersectoral linkages and health development: Case studies in India (Kerala State), Jamaica, Norway, Sri Lanka and Thailand. WHO Offset Publication No.83, Geneva: World Health Organization.

TEXTBOX 3.2. INTERSECTORAL LINKAGES IN SRI LANKA

- Focus on rice-growing peasantry, the poorest social group which led to reduction in regional disparities and inequalities
- Emphasis on self-sufficiency in food
- Development of small-scale fishing industry which caters to the poorer classes
- Satisfaction of basic needs
- Universal free education
- Food rationing system
- Emphasis on rural housing and transport

Source: Godfrey Gunatilleke (1984) Ed. Intersectoral linkages and health development: Case studies in India (Kerala State), Jamaica, Norway, Sri Lanka and Thailand. WHO Offset Publication No.83, Geneva: World Health Organization.

TEXTBOX 3.3. INTERSECTORAL LINKAGES IN THAILAND

- Growth and expansion of economy
- High rate of growth in agriculture which led to more employment and availability of food
- Diversification of crops which helped the export earnings
- Massive industrialization in the central region
- Spread of education and literacy
- Programs on basic needs
- Eradication of poverty and improvement of quality of life

Source: Godfrey Gunatilleke (1984) Ed. Intersectoral linkages and health development: Case studies in India (Kerala State), Jamaica, Norway, Sri Lanka and Thailand. WHO Offset Publication No.83, Geneva: World Health Organization.

The multi-dimensionality became more evidence based as a result of these exercises undertaken at the global level and it is now realized that universal health can be achieved only by intersectoral approaches discussed earlier in this chapter which is now being flagged as Health in All Policies. The Health in All Policy is the new thrust of the organizations such as the World Health Organization (WHO). The core of HiAP is a focus on determinants of health that can improve health but are mainly controlled by the policies of sectors other than health. Closely linked to this is the *Intersectoral action for health* which could be defined as "a coordinated action that explicitly aims to improve people's health or influence determinants of health. Intersectoral action for health is seen as central to the achievement of greater equity in health, especially where progress depends upon decisions and actions in other sectors" (Stahl et al., 2006:5).

It is a renewed attempt to grapple with ill-health through a multi-faceted, multi-pronged and intersectoral approach with recognition that health cannot be achieved or created by only Ministry of Health (Nayar, 2013). It is therefore an extension of the primary health care approach and the intersectoral vision evolved in the late 70s and early 80s. This requires bold and cooperative actions from the health sector which has to function in collaboration with other sectors often with conflicting interests and objectives.

There are several dimensions in this approach as given in the Adelaide Statement on Health in All Policies, 2010 (WHO, 2010).

In India, The *Bharat Nirman* (Development of India) and the flagship programs of the government of India demonstrate an attempt to develop an integrated approach to human development which includes health. In other words, it could be considered as an innovative approach to "Health in All" Policy. Many of these programs have direct and indirect implications for health. The following are some of the important components of the integrated package:

Rural roads
Rural housing
Drinking water
Irrigation
Rural telephony
Rural electrification
Rural employment guarantee
Education for all
Mid-day meal
Rural health
Urban renewal and urban health
Total sanitation

TEXTBOX 3.4. ADELAIDE STATEMENT ON HEALTH IN ALL POLICIES

Achieving social, economic, and environmental development
A healthy population is a key requirement for the achievement of society's goals. Reducing inequalities and the social gradient improves health and well-being for everyone.

Need for joined-up government
Governments can coordinate policy-making by developing strategic plans that set out common goals, integrated responses and increased accountability across government departments. This requires a partnership with civil society and the private sector.

Health in All Policies approach
Health in All Policies works best when:

- a clear mandate makes joined-up government an imperative
- systematic processes take account of interactions across sectors
- mediation occurs across interests
- accountability, transparency, and participatory processes are present
- engagement occurs with stakeholders outside of government
- practical cross-sector initiatives build partnerships and trust.

Source: WHO (2010): 2-3

Some of the convergent actions in India include the community insurance schemes by the Ministry of Labor and the Total Sanitation Campaign by the Ministry of Rural Development and the provision of basic amenities under Urban Renewal Mission by the Ministry of Housing and Urban Poverty Alleviation (PHFI, 2011).

Tobacco control in India has become operational with an intersectoral approach and which can evolve into one of the largest such programs in the world. An inter-ministerial task force consisting of twelve ministries spearheaded by the Ministry of Health and Family Welfare monitor the progress of FCTC implementation at the national level. Similarly, each state has a fourteen member committee and the district has an eleven-member coordination committee chaired by the District Magistrate. Coordination between sectors is reinforced by the activities of the health sector by implementing awareness-raising and sensitization activities (WHO-Government of India Biennial work plan, 2012). A sum of 33.5 million US dollars was approved for the program out of which more than 75 percent have been released. The Ministry of Health and Family Welfare funds all the intersectoral activities. Some state governments also have earmarked separate funds for tobacco control activities.

There is evidently an understanding among the policy makers regarding HiAP or a willingness to address issues from that platform given a number of policy directions at the national level. Sustaining such positive trends was a problem given the withdrawal of the state and the rise of the market. Apart from sustainability, globalization, and macro-economic scenario made it difficult to pursue a welfare agenda undertaken in the above contexts often resulting in new reform packages as in Thailand or new models to sustain the positive human development indices.

The current understanding regarding HiAP is limited but there is a consensus that it involves working across sectors which result in a healthy society. It is a strategy that allows the formulation of public policies in sectors different to the health in tandem with health services and when they are implemented these policies can correct, improve or positively influence the determinants of health.

It is important to realize that given the socio-economic conditions of the people, the state should continue to occupy a central role in the provision of care and welfare of its citizens. Apart from the state, the key driver of HiAP is the social capital especially through community level organizations including NGOs which will be examined in chapter 5. However, such actions are also not free from the same negative trends observed as part of the state-driven programs. What emerges from the experience of using social capital is that the approach has to be contextual and based on the type of barriers that exists various countries in achieving universal health. There are various patterns of discrimination that the poor go through in accessing services which cut across different states. A social capital approach may work under such conditions in which especially the women can act as pressure groups to push an intersectoral agenda and a more equitable health care. From an organizational point of view, a number of facilitating factors exist such as a commitment to decentralize both politically as well as technically. Apart from this, utilization of a community-based approach using self-help groups also could facilitate intersectoral actions and Health in All Policies provided an enabling environment such as a responsive health system is in place (see chapter 5).

CONCLUDING OBSERVATIONS

Did the reforms which were intended to grapple with the crises in health themselves lead to more crises and disorder? It appears that the so-called crisis is perennial often used as a rationale to usher in reforms of the type we critiqued in the previous sections. Although there are ideological differences in the way in which this crisis is posed in the literature, with respect to the Indian health services, the salient crisis at various points of time is the non-accessibility and non-availability of care to large sections of the people despite the fact that the poor, especially below poverty line families, prefer the government health care services (KSSP, 2006).

It is necessary to recognize that the reforms necessitated considerable tinkering with the basic structure of health services in India and changed the ethos of public provisioning of care. This also raises questions regarding obligations of the state toward their citizens, especially the poor. Needless to add, such tinkering has led to further worsening of the crises and creating more disorder at different levels which has further worsened accessibility and availability of health services. The approach of missions and visions therefore should be to create a stable and strong public sector health services which could transcend the disorder created by the reforms. The new thrust on social determinants and Health in All Policies could reinvigorate the primary health care approach and cushion the impact of reforms to some extent.

4

Centrality of Decentralization and Marginalization of the People

Decentralization in recent years has become a buzzword to make governance more acceptable to the people. From the operational point of view, decentralization has become necessary given the extreme form of centralization especially in development and welfare sectors and in some way to give a sense of people's participation in the programs evolved by the state although the paternalistic character of the state-driven programs continue to be strong. However, the legislation and decentralization initiatives of the center have led to some dilution and devolution of power to the peripheries. The Weberian justification of centralization based on cost-effectiveness, efficiency, and coverage has also been diluted which led to a sense of uncertainty and disquiet. And it was in the nineties and at the beginning of the new millennium that there was a renewed interest in decentralization which was largely due to the funding strategies and the implementation of structural adjustment and reform strategies in many countries and we find proliferating literature on different dimensions of decentralization. However, the interest has waned in recent times and the initial enthusiasm for decentralization has also reduced probably due to the lack of interest among the funding agencies such as the World Bank. There is also a trend toward re-centralization in some European countries where decentralization was implemented earlier (Saltman, 2008). A large number of state institutions are seizing the opportunity to capture financial and political powers devolved earlier to lower levels. Saltman suggests that the future will see many European countries tightening their controls over fiscal and quality matters in health care which could also weaken democratization at the regional and municipal levels.

Notwithstanding these waning interests, the role of the people in decision-making and governance is realized through processes such as decentralization and therefore with respect to health and health services, it becomes necessary to examine decentralization and its complexities in this chapter. And, in this context, there are both negative and positive forces which shape these processes at the individual, organizational, and societal levels (Huss et al., 2011). The whole approach of decentralization also has a number of tools, paraphernalia and methodologies and we may examine some of these complexities in detail while we will provide some indicative analysis in other areas. The chapter is mainly based on a review of salient literature and an iterative use of writings and papers on decentralization and allied themes and partly based on studies and fieldwork carried out for writing those papers.

A number of approaches to decentralization have been evolved, and it is interesting that they are targeted on the so-called resource-poor settings in terms of money, material and even intellectual resources! (Bossert, 1998). Rondinelli's much used categorization of decentralization process as devolution, deconcentration, delegation, and privatization was also addressed to developing countries (Rondinelli, 1983). In fact, such a categorization has been used to usher in privatization under health sector reforms as one of the strategies toward decentralization. The World Bank adopted such an approach to categorize the pattern of decentralization as political, administrative, fiscal, and market decentralization (World Bank, 2013).

Using the conventional public administration and public choice approaches along with social capital and principal agent approaches, Bossert developed an approach viz. decision space approach which is an improvement of the principal agent approach. In essence, it considers transfer of power from center (principal) to periphery (agent) but evaluates how local agents evolve innovative programs for maximizing the impact of health programs. It is clear that the managerial face of decentralization still is dominant and has influenced programs such as National Rural Health Mission. Such decentralization initiatives come out of the bureaucratic-institutional framework although they do recognize it as a complex multi-level phenomenon and they also marginalize sociopolitical processes (Saltman, Bankauskaite, Vrangbaek, 2007). There is however a realization regarding the complexity of relationships between different actors in the health system and the recognition of plurality of health organizational arrangement in the world. Any efforts to homogenize the health systems may not be successful although such a process is also on in the world. The major reason for undertaking such initiatives is to make health systems accessible to all which is assumed to have become top-down, elite-driven, and selective. Decentralization is thought to be one of the prescriptions to make it reversible by involving people in the basic functions health systems such as service provision, resource generation, financing, and stewardship (Alliance for Health Policy and Systems Research, 2004).

Many health activists initially viewed decentralization as a way to enhance community participation and empowerment. However, increasingly there is a disillusionment among them as they view the reform mode of decentralization undermine the ability of health systems to deliver their goals (Kawanga, 2005).

It is now well-accepted that universal health care is not possible without an appropriate strategy which could grapple with the institutional, technical, economic, and social dimensions of health. Essentially, decentralization of health services has to be seen as a microcosmic process of redistribution of power in the society. And this makes it ever more political. Obviously, decentralization cannot be achieved by managerial visions and homogenized models due to a number of factors (Alliance for Health Policy and Systems Research, 2004). These are:

1. The multiplicity of objectives which decentralization strategies may be used to pursue.
2. The multiplicity of forms of decentralization, and to some extent the lack of a common and consistently applied framework for defining the form of decentralization.
3. The fact that decentralization is commonly a complex and protracted reform (it is therefore often difficult to separate out the effects of decentralization from other concurrent changes in the health sector).
4. Even if common models of decentralization are adopted by several countries these models may be implemented in different ways (different sequencing of reforms, or different types of responsibilities being decentralized).

The World Bank which favors a more market-driven decentralization approach also has many caveats:

> Decentralization is not a panacea, and it does have potential disadvantages. Decentralization may not always be efficient, especially for standardized, routine, network-based services. It can result in the loss of economies of scale and control over scarce financial resources by the central government. Weak administrative or technical capacity at local levels may result in services being delivered less efficiently and effectively in some areas of the country. Administrative responsibilities may be transferred to local levels without adequate financial resources and make equitable distribution or provision of services more difficult. Decentralization can sometimes make coordination of national policies more complex and may allow functions to be captured by local elites. Also, distrust between public and private sectors may undermine cooperation at the local level. (World Bank, 2013)

INTERNATIONAL EXPERIENCES IN DECENTRALIZATION

In many parts of the world, the centralized state has been constantly challenged by rising popular movements and this process is currently witnessed in Egypt and the Middle East. However, as Pranab Bardhan points out, this has been also used as an opportunity to de-emphasize the power of over-extended and predatory state by free market economists (Bardhan, 2002). An analysis of the international experience with decentralization would help in understanding the predominant role of such market orientation and reforms in shaping the agenda. Decentralization in health care was in fact attempted in several countries, including China and Brazil, with mixed results. The Chinese decentralization led to a market orientation and a new ethos within the health services in which health facility managers generate revenue, invest the surplus in new equipment, and pay bonuses to employees. Individuals and institutions now give priority to earning money. This form of decentralization was successful in the penetration of market into the health service system while maintaining it as a non-political entity (Bloom and Xingyuan, 1997). Although decentralization had become an official policy in Brazil after the fall of the military regime in of 1964-1985, there was a gap between the type of decentralization called for in the national constitution and the de-concentration actually implemented (Araujo and Luiz, 1997). This gap is explained by Brazil's centralist tradition, resistance at the national level, and the weaknesses of local governments.

In Zambia, inter-regional inequalities increased during the decentralization process, when wealthier districts and hospitals in those districts could raise more funds and were able to draw key staff away from the less wealthy areas by offering them better terms and conditions (Standing, 1997). In Senegal, where high levels of political, financial, and managerial devolution to community health committees were achieved, the cost of prenatal check-ups and the cost of maternal deliveries increased. As a result, health services utilization substantially decreased among mothers and infants (Standing, 1997). A number of other constraints have been observed in the decentralized health delivery system in Latin America, as well as in African countries, such as Kenya, Sudan, and Tanzania (Collins and Green, 1994). These include inadequate number of trained staff, inadequate financial resources, and poor administrative capabilities.

In the USA, the era of decentralization—new federalism—led to Medicare cuts and massive restructuring of health care by the private market (Estes and Linkins, 1997). It caused a debate whether devolution reform could achieve national goals other than those related to a reduced federal role in domestic health and social policy. It has been pointed out that the dominant structural, economic, and political interests operating at the federal level are not likely to be challenged by the fragmented and diverse interest groups for the poor at the state and local level. With decentralized policy making, those who are well-off, best funded, and best organized corner most of the benefits. Given limited taxing capacity and fiscal resources of the states and localities, social services faced severe stress and therefore, problems of access to care became more acute.

Sri Lanka with a long history of political decentralization also attempted the reform model of decentralization under external pressure although it did not result in much organizational delegation or devolution of power to the lower levels (Attanayake, 2001). Probably, the disparities between provinces with respect to resource allocation, access to care, and quality of care, etc. had eased out largely due to the primary health care policy adopted by the state than decentralization strategies which again points out the irrelevance of managerial decentralization under a reform package.

THE INDIAN CASE OF DECENTRALIZATION

Since independence in 1947, India has been witness to several phases of decentralization. From the initial token support to the process, decentralization became constitutionally sacrosanct in the nineties. In between, there were also attempts to marginalize the role of local governments by bypassing them through the delivery of developmental programs directly to the villages. Multitudes of government committees have examined and suggested measures to strengthen the *panchayati raj* institutions (local self-government) since independence. The local governments were apparently rejuvenated by the constitutional amendments in 1992 although constitutional support and legislative amendments or setting up of governing structures are not sufficient conditions for achieving such goals (Mathew, 1998; Kothari, 1996). Many state governments in India have not completed the follow-up process even after two decades of initiating the constitutional changes and elections are not held regularly for the local bodies. It is often argued that inadequate political participation and inequality often exist together and initiatives which enhance democracy at the grass-roots may help in wiping out such handicaps (Dreze and Sen, 2002). However, as Dreze and Sen argue, mere rejuvenation of democratic institutions does not necessarily lead to participation of the people unless some of the determining factors such as inequalities are addressed. Due to the technical nature of health services, this is more complex and challenging as the technical sphere has to negotiate the social spaces riddled with poverty and inequality. Apart from this, the foundations of health services, viz. the health institutions, the functionaries and their involvement in the delivery of health care and the involvement of the people in the management of health services and above all, equity in care all are also important for developing a democratic health institution. It is evident that it is not a simple unidimensional devolution but a multidimensional and multifaceted political and technical democratization which could be effective. Perhaps, it is this complexity which could have been responsible for the mixed result of success and failures as decentralization is often conceived within a framework of social engineering. The two prerequisites for decentralized governance are an appropriate institutional structure and an environment conducive for carrying out the functions (Aziz, 2000). Aziz identifies number of parameters for the normative model of decentralization under each of these prerequisites. For the institutional framework, the following are needed:

1. An institution to articulate and represent the needs of the people
2. An administration which can carry out these functions and implement local level plans.
3. A data collection machinery to collect data on the basis of which plans and programs can be evolved.

These institutional prerequisites function in an environment which has the following attributes:

1. an equitable representation of interest groups in decision-making
2. people's participation in the planning process
3. political and financial autonomy
4. presence of competent experts for evolving technically sound plans
5. a satisfactory coordination with the higher levels in the tier system of governance
6. close association with the governance and the civil society.

The decentralization initiatives undertaken in different countries and in the states of India have to be judged against these attributes.

As mentioned in the beginning, decentralization is a meeting ground for the people and the state and it also has been one of the essential ingredients of health sector reforms and therefore an analysis of the dynamics is a part of any critical reflections on the role of the state and the people in health services development. Similar to health services development as discussed in the previous two chapters, decentralization has also been instrumentalized and bureaucratized to a large extent. In other words, role of the people in shaping health services has been marginalized through this instrumentalization as well as by the dominance of a reform agenda despite exceptions in some states. This chapter is based largely on the international experience of decentralization and the experience in some selected states in India and especially the state of Kerala. It also attempts to reflect on some of the conceptual and methodological issues both from the point of view of considering decentralization as essentially political and from the reform view of considering it in discrete and disaggregate terms as fiscal, managerial, and political.

The Indian initiative on decentralization did not primarily emerge as a response to reform package but as a part of the political expedience felt by the ruling elite (Nayar, 1998). Therefore, the content of decentralization initiative initially was much more political than managerial. It was also due to a growing recognition that regional disparities and inequalities have widened despite national planning (Mathur, 1998). The 73rd and the 74th amendments of the Indian constitution and the consequent acts in the states heralded a new era in decentralized governance by making elections mandatory and preventing state governments from superseding the institutions for indefinite periods. Under this act, a set of items were entrusted with the local self-governments which comprise health and sanitation including hospitals, primary health centers, and dispensaries, family welfare, housing, drinking water, etc. (Government of India, 1993). These institutions have to receive adequate funds to carry out these functions, including grants from the state governments and a share of certain taxes. This would be in addition to the revenue that the councils were allowed to raise and retain with them. Notwithstanding the legislation to facilitate decision-making at lower levels, the degree of political commitment continue to determine whether or not such institutions can become effective levels of governance with enlarged participation of the local communities (Satishchandran, 1994).

CONCEPTUAL CONFUSIONS

Decentralization is normally understood in relation to power and resources. However, in recent years a number of redefinitions have been attempted especially by the World Bank. As a parallel process, decentralization has in recent years become a tool for ushering in a neo-liberal developmental agenda. This marks a clear shift in the conceptualization of decentralization, moving away from a political process to the level of total withdrawal of the state. The World Bank, which has been promoting neo-liberal economic packages as a part of the structural adjustment programs, as mentioned earlier has come out with new conceptualizations. The World Bank in its conceptualization has placed political decentralization along with administrative, fiscal, and market forms of decentralization. According to the Bank, the most complete forms of decentralization from a government's perspective are privatization and deregulation because they shift responsibility for functions from the public to the private sector. This not only underemphasizes the political and democratic content of the process but also promotes privatization as the complete form of decentralization.

On the other hand, there are also confusions regarding administrative and political forms of decentralization. This has implications for health services as the dichotomy between technical decisions and political control lead to conflicts and confusions. Some of these have been documented after the experience of decentralization in Karnataka and during the people's planning process in Kerala (Satishchandran, 1993; Nayar, 2001). These include those related to administrative control of resources as well as that of personnel especially at the lower levels. For instance, in Karnataka, there was considerable misunderstanding among the different segments of the government regarding personnel issues such as transfers, disciplinary control, and their administrative boundaries. The Maharashtra experience shows increasing groupism on the basis of parochial considerations, failure of panchayats (village-level institution under local self-government) to harness new resources, overdependence on the government funds, etc. (Rao, 1994). The major problem in West Bengal was with regard to the allocation of resources. For schemes implemented by the local governments, funds are received in numerous unpredictable installments throughout the year, making rational implementation of programs extremely difficult (Mukherjee and Bandhopadhyay, 1995). In Madhya Pradesh, in spite of considerable support from the state government, the panchayats faced double-edged hostility from the district bureaucracy which feared loss of its power and the elected representatives at the higher levels who tend to see panchayat representatives as competitors in their local political arena (Jaffri, 2001).

The conflict between the professional and the political leadership is one of the challenges in the decentralization process. The existing health personnel do not participate at the planning process as they are largely perceived as executives. It is possible to identify a number of conflicts between the *panchayats* and the state government. The state government evolves the major chunk of the programs that are handed down to the *panchayats* for implementation. With regard to health services, a number of areas where conflicts can surface could be identified. These include: (i) drug supply which is controlled by the state; (ii) recruitment of staff, service matters including leave; and (iii) allocation and proportion of funds for need-based and other programs (Nayar, 2001). Another area of possible conflict is between centrally sponsored schemes and the programs evolved by the state. The responsibility for implementing centrally sponsored schemes is with the *panchayats*. In effect, the negative features of the vertical programs would continue to affect health in spite of elaborately prepared programs at the local levels. In Kerala, although recent initiatives indicate a progressive move toward a political form of decentralization, there are still some resistance at the upper levels, especially from the state-level political leaders and bureaucrats. There have been also confusions about the extent of power, resources and responsibilities to be transferred to the lower levels as bureaucrats and politicians normally do not like their power to be curtailed. Jaffri points out that there are sharply contrasting groups in the arena of *panchayats* in Madhya Pradesh—the traditionally influential and entrenched representatives and the other is the new entrants (Jaffri, 2001). The conflict between the two sections was on the expected lines of caste and class background. All these confusions and conflicts not only result in a degree of uncertainty regarding decentralization but they also strengthen the forces of centralization to some extent.

It is not only forces of centralization that the exploited classes have to counter but even the techno-managerial forms of decentralization in the era of structural adjustment. In these difficult times, a vision which places faith on people's power gets marginalized. It appears that there are no options available to the poor and working classes in this country against the onslaught of neo-liberal agenda. However, some states like Kerala have been experimenting and exploring new ways to intervene in the available spaces to bring back people's power to the center stage as against the ruthless techno-managerial visions.

Nationally, decentralization has been visible in multitudes of micro-level processes which include operational, financial and political dimensions cutting across different ideological strains. These include people's planning which is the most radical among the decentralization initiatives; public-private partnerships in maternity care; contracting of private specialist doctors in the primary health center; formation of quasi government societies, etc.

PEOPLE'S POWER AND THE STATE

A brief examination of the process of decentralization attempted in Kerala will enable us to understand how an effort was made through a series of programs to ensure democratic, participatory, and justice-oriented development in the emerging world order under the name of people's planning, one of the much publicized and eulogized mega decentralization project. This was one which was not only "venerated by all but was practiced as well." The people's plan sailed well as long as there was political support for it and it started sinking when the left-front government, the originator left the scene. However, given the democratic approach to its conceptualization, planning, implementation and monitoring of the process, it is very important to understand the dynamics which were in operation at the micro level. This is especially so since the program may disappear in to the annals of history.

The Planning Board of Kerala tried to implement the integrated people's planning in four stages (Government of Kerala, 1997):

1. At stage one, resource maps were prepared in order to understand water and other resources in each plot of land. This was undertaken by voluntary workers and local level experts.
2. At the second stage, studies on socioeconomic status, problems in the village, institutions, and history was attempted to provide a human dimension to developmental programs. This was conducted by a survey of all the households in the village.
3. At the third stage, the developmental programs were evolved, using the data from resource maps and socio-economic survey. Two types of programs were identified: one which can be implemented with the available data sources and the other which requires further studies.
4. At the last stage, the development programs were given the final shape ensuring at the same time their sustainability and potential of ensuring continuous participation of the people. It was also hoped that, along with the need-based programs, the schemes that have been handed over to the village councils and municipalities could also be successfully and effectively implemented through this process.

The entire process of implementation also had many activities, such as meetings of village and municipal ward, developmental seminars, formation of working groups for assessing developmental programs evolved by this process, state-level working groups, and training at different levels.

If we examine the content of "health" in the above mentioned process of decentralization and people's planning, we could identify a number of weaknesses. Although the health status of Kerala had been acclaimed all over the world, reports had predicted that that it stood on a weak base (Ekbal and Ramankutty, 1996). The public health system in the state had collapsed and the government hospitals had lost their credibility. About 60 percent of the hospitals and health workers, including physicians remain in the private sector, inaccessible to 30–40 percent of the people. It is in this context that the implementation of people's planning was considered as a remedy for overcoming the crises in the health service system. The issues of quality and accessibility of health services had to be kept in mind in the process of decentralization. The health status in Kerala was a major conundrum in which it was pointed out that despite an epidemiological transition there exist several paradoxes including a paradox of low mortality and high morbidity (Panikkar and Soman, 1984). The epidemiological pattern with respect to the Kerala society was extremely complex. The morbidity at that point of time was broadly similar to that of India as a whole with respect to communicable diseases. Therefore, in any decentralized health care delivery system, there was a need to recognize and resolve such paradoxes and complexities.

A content analysis of the themes identified by six village councils while evolving projects in health showed that they fall into several categories. The identified programs included sanitation, expansion of indigenous systems of medicine, removal of garbage and waste, up-gradation of services in the primary health centers, health education, and health camps, etc. (Nayar, 2001). This means that preventive aspects had been given emphasis by the people, which could be considered a positive step. However, the crises in the health service system in Kerala were largely in relation to the delivery of communicable disease control programs and the supply of drugs and quality of curative care. It appeared that in the initial phases of people's planning these aspects were not covered. On the other hand, some of the preventive programs identified by the people did not get sufficient attention of the health services as they fell outside their ambit or because of the costs of implementing some of these programs.

A study of people's planning in Kerala by Jose George reported that the decentralized planning resulted in significant increase in the funds earmarked and spent for the scheduled castes and scheduled tribes (George, 2003). During the people's campaign and afterwards, the plan allocations for the weaker sections went up by 30 to 40 percent. Gender justice was also declared as one of the important objectives of the people's campaign. A special Women's Component Plan with 10 percent outlay was also set up apart from fulfilling the criteria of one-third reservation of seats. It is observed that elected women representatives were better qualified than men although many of them had to bear the triple burden of public office, income earning, and domestic duties. The study also found that decentralization of corruption to the village level, widespread nepotism and the dominance of contractors were minimal and more due to inexperience and haste rather than planned corruption. The unholy contractor-engineer-politician nexus was broken in many *panchayats*. As the campaign progressed the quantum of such incidents came down. The neighborhood groups and the *grama sabhas* (village councils) performed as a check on these imbalances. Regular meetings of these institutions helped in reducing corruption and irregularities.

The case study provides evidence that caste and class divisions at the villages need not be a constraint for participatory planning as it is normally believed. The success is attributed to an effective leadership at the village level, mass mobilization above party lines and a political will at the top. The two institutions which played a significant role in the mobilization as well as in sustaining the momentum are the neighborhood groups (*ayalkoottams*) and the *grama sabha*.

CONFLICTS AND CONTRADICTIONS IN PEOPLE'S PLANNING: LESSONS FOR DECENTRALIZED HEALTH CARE

It is possible to say, notwithstanding the considerable advantages of people's planning, that resource constraints and multiple authorities will continue to plague the effectiveness of the identified programs. Secondly, the type of programs which do not intervene into the core area of health and health services could result in the continued supremacy of medical bureaucracy in the villages. To some extent, the type of programs identified by the people portend demystification of health but at the same time it is also necessary to think in terms of interventions which make the health service system more vibrant and efficient.

A more vibrant and responsive health service system resulting from people's direct participation in the planning process was not realized, as a number of conflicts and gaps which were discernible posed constraints on the effective implementation of a much appreciated legislation. Based on the content analysis and the field work undertaken in the villages, the following conflicts and gaps could be identified (Nayar, 2001).

1. An understanding of gaps between the need-based programs identified and actually felt need on the one hand and those between need-based programs and the epidemiological need would further help in consolidating the effectiveness such initiatives. This is essential for taking forward the process of democratization of health services and the approach of primary health care.
2. The second level of conflict is between the professional and the political leadership at the village level. The existing health personnel did not participate at the policy planning stage, nor did they participate at the project preparatory stage. They were also largely excluded during the participatory training programs. In short, doctors and other health workers were supposed to implement the evolved programs without their participation during formulation. The total exclusion of health service system thus raised the issue of new conflicts in the villages which continue even in present times.

3. A number of conflicts between the village councils and the state government could also be identified. The state government evolved the major chunk of the programs which were handed down to the lower levels for implementation. With regard to health services, many areas where conflicts become discernible could be identified. These included: (a) drug supply which is controlled by the state, (b) recruitment of staff, service matters including leave, etc., and (c) allocation and proportion of funds for need-based and other programs.
4. Another possible conflict which was prominent was between centrally sponsored schemes and the programs evolved by the state. It needs to be pointed out that the centrally sponsored schemes remain as they are and the lower levels of governance are bound by them. In effect, the negative features of the vertical programs continue to affect health even if programs are evolved by the people.
5. As mentioned earlier, like all other earlier initiatives on devolution of political and financial powers to the lower levels, Kerala had also witnessed a kind of resistance at the upper levels, especially the state level political leaders and bureaucrats. There also exists widespread perception among the upper echelons of the bureaucracy that the lower-level functionaries and politicians are incapable of handling programs including finances. The government need to give due attention to overhaul village and municipal laws to make the devolution more effective.
6. Another level of conflict emerged within the health service system regarding the form of preventive and curative programs. While most of the evolved programs were preventive programs, there was utter lack of clarity and total confusion regarding the role of health services in this process.
7. Needless to say, all the conflicts inherent in an agrarian society were also visible at the village level, which could ultimately threaten the sustainability of the programs.

People's planning and the process of decentralization in the Indian state of Kerala may be considered as an expression of democratic rights of the people in an effort to counter the onslaught of globalization and centralization of governance. The type of decentralization attempted in Kerala, in which power and resources were transferred to lower levels of governance and different sections of the population were involved in planning, distinguished it from other such attempts elsewhere in the country and in other countries. To that extent, it could be considered as a lesson and a model for those countries undergoing structural adjustment. Since people themselves were planning for health care and the agenda was not imposed from above, it could be effectively used as a tool for strengthening primary health care through which communicable diseases control programs could be effectively implemented under people's supervision. The experiment as expected had a mixed face but it has been pointed out by scholars that it has not been an unmitigated failure either (Das, 2000). There have been a number of cases when panchayats developed programs according to the visions of people's planning and brought about changes in the society.

The Kerala example could be used to highlight the social and technical dimensions of the process of decentralization, which was largely visualized as a legislative exercise. The effectiveness of participatory development could be enhanced if such dimensions could be given adequate importance and the conflicts and contradictions resolved. The Kerala experiment could succeed to some extent due to the fact that the existing power structures were more conducive to at least develop a sense of participation by all sections although political cleavages and competitive welfarism often frustrated complete participation (Bardhan, 2002).

One could state that with the exception of some states including Kerala, decentralization in India in terms of implementing efficient public health interventions, increasing transparency, accountability and efficiency and integrated delivery with people's participation has been a failure. In one of the earliest reviews, it has been pointed out that the pressure for greater autonomy is not coming from below as the general perception of the people about the panchayats as a powerless body and therefore inappropriate to handle their problems (Mahipal, 2004). It is generally felt that the *panchayati raj* institutions will remain subjugated and controlled by the state and central governments as there is lack of commitment to devolve power by the political parties despite much celebrated constitutional amendments.

THE MANAGERIAL FACE OF DECENTRALIZATION IN HEALTH

As against a people-oriented and politically loaded decentralization, the present decentralization strategies are managerial for implementing a packaged health program in villages. The National Rural Health Mission (NRHM) is perhaps the first program in India to use professional managers to implement health programs. Most of these managers thus employed by the quasi-government set-up at the district level are young management graduates of some management institutes often with half-baked understanding of district health infrastructure. Mostly, these reforms were a boon for the managers and a bane for the health service system in India. It need to be underscored that conventional management strategies and the new public management

(NPM) churned out of market-driven mold and produced in management schools often are inadequate as there is a larger component of epidemiology and social science factors which determine health conditions and utilization of health services. Health services need to be visualized differently from other consumption items mass produced in factories. In recent times, efforts are also on to develop the new public management (NPM) which we referred to in chapter 3 to hospital management as well under the guise of granting autonomy to public hospitals (Saltman, Duran, and Dubois, 2011). In India, efforts such as creation of hospital management committees with participation of stakeholders have been tried out without much success. The creation of medical corporations such as in Tamil Nadu has led to some success in the creation of more accessible services and availability of drugs. However, this is largely due to the existence of a strong public sector health network prior to the implementation of reforms rather than the impact of reforms (Sigamani, 2005). In many states, the public hospitals remain as inhospitable as before despite user fees and management committees!

Under National Rural Health Mission (NRHM), decentralization was attempted by forming the Village Health and Sanitation Committees and also by developing a system of governance and planning which was district-centered. This is probably the first time that the cleavages between centralization and decentralization were reduced by apportioning the decision-making regarding allocation, policy formulation, and implementation between the center and states. Such a process could have led to an element of recentralization as well. Evidently, the Common Review Mission carried out in 2010 pointed out that the district planning efforts have considerably weakened in many states with the district planning process reduced to filling up template forms (Government of India, 2011). The district planning was meant to facilitate, 1) infrastructure development, 2) imparting of skilled training, 3) procurement and logistics, 4) technical resource centers, 5) community-oriented resource centers, etc. With the exception of Kerala, none of the states have these five components in place. Kerala and Tamil Nadu stand out in having procurement units in place. The Common Review Mission report identified that the district plans were not used for the allocation of funds which result in these plans being reduced to routine activities. It was found that in the fifth year of NRHM, there was fatigue as well as cynicism associated with the district planning activities. The Village Health and Sanitation Committees (VHSC) although formed in many states, they are poorly functional and there is lack of clarity in their mandates. Exceptions are Assam, Maharashtra, Kerala and Odisha. The representation of marginalized sections in these committees is also absent. The involvement of *panchayati raj* institutions in health is also extremely sloppy and notional in many states except in Kerala as health often is not a tangible entity for the political leaders.

INSTITUTIONAL AND COMMUNITY-LEVEL INNOVATIONS

One of the most important outcomes of devolution of power to the lower levels is the process of autonomy created by such initiatives which expresses itself in innovations. These can be basically categorized into two types—institutional innovations and community-level innovations. The National Rural Health Mission although has a larger paternalistic program components, it has also facilitated some degree of autonomy with respect to administrative and technical decision-making. Most of these need to be evaluated with respect to their epidemiological and administrative soundness. Some of the innovations that we discuss below have emerged from both institutions as well as the community. Although community-led initiatives are very few, most of them are community facilitated or driven or the ones which are necessitated by community demands.

A number of institutional and community-level innovations have taken place in states which happened partly due to the activities spurred by the mission mode and partly due to the decentralization initiatives (Nayar, 2014).

Maharastra is a state which is closer to achieving the Millennium Development Goals. One of the salient initiatives to bring the tribal population closer to the health services was undertaken in the Amravati district of the state. This was to help the excluded tribal population of the district to access various services of the public sector health services by providing a counselor who speaks the language of the tribal population. This helped to reduce the cultural gap between health institutions and the people. The state's nutrition mission was also considered to be an innovation which helped in reducing the malnutrition among tribal children in the Marathwada region. This was made possible by commitment and sustained efforts initiated by the official machinery and especially by the mission leadership (*Hindustan Times*, It can happen in India, December 20, 2011).

Kerala is one of the few states with almost 100 percent institutional deliveries, the highest maternal and child health outcomes as well as the first state to achieve MDG targets. The current thrust on institutional deliveries to achieve better maternal health is based on evidence from Kerala where it is assumed that the institutional deliveries have contributed to bringing down MMR. Despite the achievement of such high rates of institutional delivery and health outcomes, the state has evolved a number of innovations to bring the women closer to the health services. Some of the innovative approaches undertaken in Kerala are as follows:

Kerala has evolved a State Women's Policy in 2009. The policy recognizes the multi-focused and multi-dimensional inputs and initiatives required for enabling women. There were initiatives to empower women's access to maternal and child care through directly enabling the ASHA workers who are also members of women's self-help groups known as *kudumbasree*. They have been successful in facilitating women's access right from the prenatal stage including access to the entry point (reception) to the labor rooms as well as postnatal care. The self-help groups are also involved in preparing nutritious food packets for the *anganwadi* under Integrated Child Development Scheme (see box 4.1).

Unlike many other states, even the comprehensive insurance scheme (CHIS/RSBY) implemented in Kerala resulted in strengthening public sector hospitals and the maternity care which is utilized by the poor. The insurance scheme incorporated maternity care for reimbursement of costs. Many initiatives have also been taken to improve the immunization status in the

TEXTBOX 4.1. ROLE OF WOMEN'S SELF-HELP GROUPS IN NUTRITION OF CHILDREN AND MOTHERS

Women self help groups help the local self government institutions as well as local level health service institutions like primary health centers in carrying out sanitation measures in the locality especially during the monsoon season like distribution of bleaching powder, finding out mosquito breeding sites, etc. But very interestingly one of the innovations in Maternal and Child Health program in Kerala is the distribution of 'AMRUTHAM' (a powdered mix of Ragi, Wheat, Sugar and Soya bean) supplied by a unit of *kudumbasree* (self-help groups). The production of *Amrutham* is supported by Integrated Child Development Sscheme (ICDS) to improve maternal and child health in Kerala and it is distributed to the beneficiaries through *anganwadi* (ICDS) workers and ASHA workers in the locality.

There are 28 such units working in Kannur district of Kerala. It is distributed in such a manner that each child will get 6 packets in a month (I packet contains 563 grams) from 6 months to 3 years. Our primary survey reveals that one such unit in Korom *panchayat* of Kannur district supplies this product in the above mentioned manner to 970 children in the Payyanur municipality, 300 children in the Kadannappilly *panchayat*, 500 children in Cheruthazham *panchayat* and 350 children in Karivellur *panchayat*. Thus altogether this single unit of self-help group produces 12,720 packets in a month for serving 2120 children in nearby areas of this *panchayat*.

state. Immunization sessions are organized in the remote areas giving special attention to tribal, coastal, and urban slums. In the low coverage areas, immunization activities are strengthened with the help of NGOs and private institutions.

As opposed to this best-case scenario, *Jharkhand* continues to share a number of characteristics with other backward states of India such as high infant mortality, low immunization of children and expectant mothers, high mortality due to infectious and contagious diseases, high maternal mortality, and low institutional delivery. Reviews and studies of NRHM in Jharkhand have shown that the process of decentralization, responsiveness to local needs, paradigm shift in health system management and availability of untied funds have improved the facilities and their credibility among the people. Earlier, there existed ignorance, inhibitions and lack of awareness on issues of MCH, reproductive health and rights, adolescent reproductive and sexual health, abortion, etc. among the population. Gradually with intensive interventions adopting comprehensive IEC/ BCC strategies there is increased awareness and articulation on these issues. This has been facilitated through the concerted involvement of NGOs and civil society organizations. Today there is a receptive community and a wider platform for dissemination on reproductive issues and beyond. Setting-up of Sahiya Resource Center is one innovation that has helped this process of community mobilization. It was evident from the fieldwork that the women activists can positively channelize the responses of the people (see box 42). Unfortunately, such activities have not resulted in an increase in institutional deliveries and the state continues to remain at the bottom of the ladder. In *Uttarakhand*, a hill state of India, interviews with Accredited Social Health Activists (ASHA) revealed that due to absence of roads in the higher altitudes, ambulances cannot reach their villages. This disabled the pregnant woman to reach any hospital for delivery. Some success stories from districts like Barav saw the Village Health and Sanitation Committee (VHSC) making a *palki* (a stretcher like carrier) to enable the lady in labor to reach till the main road up till where the ambulance could travel. Such culturally appropriate innovations for transport are a small step toward developing a vibrant MCH care in rural areas.

Bringing the excluded tribal population is another major challenge for the JSY program. In the tribal dominated state of *Odishsa*, maternity waiting homes (MWH) are constructed in most remote tribal block of several districts (Government of Odisha, undated). This has helped in developing positive attitudes to institutional deliveries. The MWH function like a platform for the expectant mothers to come before hand, which is to be established in the mid-way to the institution. Due to extreme poverty, women cannot afford to stay outside before delivery and such homes provide a social support to them.

The ASHAs have been able to also facilitate immunization among children. Similar to many other states such as Jharkhand and Uttarakhand, geographical accessibility is a major problem in Odisha.

In *Rajasthan*, the awareness level of *Janani Suraksha Yojana* is as high as 95 percent (UNFPA, 2009). The state had evolved a program called "panchamrit" in 2006 in which fixed day and fixed site outreach services to reach child and maternal care to families living below poverty line in each village of the state. The focus is also for covering far flung and tribal dominated districts by providing six components such as immunization, elimination of micro-nutrient deficiency, ensuring safe motherhood, and ensuring healthy newborn. Such an innovation could have led to some positive impacts in terms reducing lack of accessibility to excluded and marginalized populations. Rajasthan also experimented with a program called "Parinche" under NRHM which aimed at empowering rural communities through provision of public health programs in sanitation, nutrition, and communicable diseases through a female community health worker.

Madhya Pradesh is one of the states which has evolved a draft health policy which purports to reduce inequities in health care including gender inequities (Government of Madhya Pradesh, 2012). The *Janani Sehyogi Yojana* in Madhya Pradesh is another innovation which is meant to improve neonatal and maternal care in rural areas for the families living below poverty line by providing emergency care as well as qualitative curative support to new born children and pre- and postnatal care to women (Government of Madhya Pradesh, 2012a). The *Janani Express Yojana* provides transport facilities to pregnant women to the health facility. Apart from factors such as provision of transport to pregnant women, payment of cash incentives to mothers and ASHA, involvement of private sector, etc., community mobilization has facilitated an increased awareness and an increase in institutional deliveries in Madhya Pradesh, Rajasthan, and Odisha. More than three-fourths of the mothers in Madhya Pradesh, Rajasthan, Odisha, and Bihar knew that the health facilities are open round the clock for delivery services (UNFPA, 2009).

The state of *West Bengal* has initiated the "ayushmati" scheme which engaged the private sector in providing essential and emergency obstetric care to the below poverty line and scheduled caste/scheduled tribe families. The cost of this service would be borne by the government. Qualitative field work conducted in a district revealed that although the services have improved tremendously, there are problems in disbursal of payment, lack of transportation, lack of proper SC/ST, and BPL certificates, etc. are some of the constraints in the program.

Chattisgarh is one of the states which initiated people-friendly health services even before the implementation of NRHM. The *Mitanin* program which is the pre-cursor of the Accredited Social Health Activist (ASHA) program originated in this state. Evaluation of *Mitanin* program shows that it has been more effective compared to the ASHA in other states in terms of reaching the pregnant women, newborn and infants in aspects like newborn care, child feeding practices, diarrhea management, etc. (European Union and Government of Chattisgarh, 2011). This could be attributed, as evident from the evaluation, to their involvement in the community and their commitment to serve the people. The evaluation also shows that the *Mitanins* have been able to increase awareness, help in empowerment of women, facilitate institutional deliveries, and increase the rates of immunization. The state also evolved a scheme to place health into *Panchayat's* agenda named the *Swasth Panchayat* scheme. This is a program to support local health planning and to enhance decentralization in health. An indicator based health and human development index has been prepared for all *Panchayats* of the state that is hamlet-centered so as to capture the intra-*panchayat* variations. The *panchayats* are also encouraged to develop village health plans through people's participation (Government of Chattisgarh, 2012).

In *Gujarat*, the State Policy for Gender Equity (GEP) is formulated with a vision to safeguard women and create awareness, fostering well-being and security of women in the state. The Gujarat government has evolved a number of packages and schemes for the overall health and well-being female children and women. In health, the *Chiranjeevi Yojana* implemented by the government of Gujarat is aimed to encourage families below poverty line (BPL) to improve access to institutional delivery in partnership with the private sector. The scheme also provides for financial support to the accompanying person for loss of wages (Government of Gujarat, 2012).

The Fourth Common Review Mission (CRM) reported that innovations like boat clinics in some states like Kerala and Assam have helped to enhance accessibility to care in remote areas cut-off by water bodies. The palliative care evolved in Kerala is also an innovation mentioned by the Common Review Mission (Government of India, 2011).

METHODOLOGICAL CHALLENGES

In this backdrop, it is indeed challenging to study the process of decentralization especially given the conflicts and confusions that have arisen in recent years. One of the limitations is the lack of existing studies as the new process of decentralization is still in its infancy and forces are trying to thwart the considerable political fallout due to giving power to the lower levels. This necessitates an exploratory design for the studies. This is probably the first challenge in the methodological approach. Secondly, the reason for adopting an exploratory design, apart from the lack of existing studies, is the absence of the process of decentralization in an explicit form in some of the states which makes the researcher wonder about the viability of proceeding with the studies. Therefore, the challenge is to understand the process as it exists, identify the gaps, probe deeper, and undertake case studies to develop assumptions and hypotheses for future studies. More specifically, the methodological approach to decentralization and health has to focus on two issues: the dynamic relations between technical and political spheres and; the process and dynamics of decentralization.

Technical and Political Sphere

Understanding the conflict between the technical (aspects related to the health service system) and the political spheres is one of the most important methodological challenges. This is because of a number of reasons. Firstly, there exist considerable legal and administrative initiatives for decentralization within the political sphere while there are only marginal efforts to decentralize the health services system. Most of the decision-making within the health services system is still concentrated at the district level and above. Any efforts to understand the linkages between the political and the technical spheres have to consider this.

Secondly, the conflict between the two spheres may not be revealed or may be captured only superficially in survey research as both the actors within the spheres tend to deny any such conflicts while responding to survey questions. Only adequate rapport and an in-depth probing would capture the entire gamut of conflicts and confusions between the two spheres.

Thirdly, even within the respective spheres, there exist ambiguities regarding the process of decentralization. The technical sphere tend to consider this as a political initiative while the political sphere would like to believe that without corresponding decentralization within the health service system, it is possible to have the administrative control over the technical staff such as doctors and health workers. The doctors and health workers normally eschew and resist any control by elected representatives at the lower levels, especially regarding matters related to their service. This is one of the reasons for the negligible impact of political decentralization (however limited it be) on health care. Any study on decentralization and health care has to grapple with these complexities that exist especially in the Indian context.

Process and Dynamics

Another aspect which merits methodological attention is the process and the dynamics of decentralization. The "process" of decentralization refers to an examination of the historical, legislative, policy, and administrative dimensions. It also needs to examine how the functionaries both in the technical and political spheres perceive decentralization as it can be assumed that their worldviews—perceptions, views, attitudes, and approaches influence it to considerable extent. Unfortunately, there are very few studies on these issues.

The "dynamics" of decentralization includes a number of political, social, and cultural variables. Prominent among them are the gender differentials among the functionaries, caste and class considerations, and political affiliations. The study of dynamics should also include the social dimensions in relation to the village community, such as the caste-class-gender issues, political behavior, needs of the community, etc.

It is evident that a complex framework is necessary in order to bring out some of the complexities within the process and dynamics of decentralization, to grapple with the conceptual issues, and to understand the different levels of the administrative structure. This does not mean that any single study should or can investigate the entire gamut of the process and dynamics. The need for an *iterative* process which moves from simple level exploratory approaches to more complex and abstract constructions is to be recognized.

From a methodological point of view, a study of decentralization and its linkages with health services is most challenging. It is challenging because of the conceptual confusions with regard to the process of decentralization, the dichotomy that exists between health services and the *panchayti raj* institutions, and above all the slipshod nature of implementation of decentralization in several states of India despite lofty ideals and crafty legislation. It is also challenging because of the complexity that exists within health services as well as within the *panchayati raj* institutions. The impact on delivery of health services may be easier to assess compared to health outcomes as there are considerable influence of confounding variables. However, there are studies which report reduction in inequity over selected indicators with regard to infrastructure, utilization, and outcomes of health although they do not claim to impact analysis studies (Mishra, 2011). Despite these problems, there is a need to document the existing status to understand the features, trends, extent of problems, and the prospects of decentralization in India with respect health and health services (James, 2007).

We found that health services occupied the least priority among the elected representatives at the lower levels of governance. They are still controlled by the bureaucracy. As mentioned earlier, bureaucrats consider elected representatives, functionaries, and the people incompetent to handle issues related to development and health. This results in conflicts at the lower levels. Most of the money is spent on salaries, centrally evolved programs etc. Local level planning, when undertaken, are limited to tangible programs such as construction of buildings etc. rather than health programs. Coordination between rural self-government and official agencies occur only in intensive drives like pulse-polio program. We also found that even in this conventional form of political decentralization, there have been confusions about the extent of power, resources, and responsibilities to be transferred to the lower levels as bureaucrats and politicians normally do not like their power to be curtailed. We argue that these confusions work as channels to usher in the neo-liberal packages in decentralization. The actions which are projected as decentralization facilitate deemphasizing the state. Some of the initiatives that we observe under the National Rural Health Mission such as the increasing role of private sector indicate such a trend. It is under such conditions that an alternative need-based focused social action is necessary especially in vulnerable states of India.

CONCLUDING OBSERVATIONS: FOCUSED GROUP ACTIONS AND COLLECTIVE MOBILIZATION

The main thrust of this chapter was to highlight the forms of decentralization especially salient for health services. It could identify the extreme instrumental framework pursued while attempting to decentralize power which is essentially meant to ameliorate the problems of the poor. It also showed the complexity and confusions that galore while thrusting such a process on the social space. The different typologies of decentralization witnessed in India range from purely managerial forms such as in National Rural Health Mission and instrumentalized approaches such as the political decentralization attempted in various states to more inclusive, comprehensive, culturally acceptable and progressive approaches. Among the more progressive decentralization initiatives in India, the People's Planning in Kerala which was a state-initiated program and the *Dalli Rajhara* experience in Chattisgarh which was a people's movement are contrasting models for collective mobilization. The latter, especially has evolved out of people's own response to long history of oppression and resistance although such movements may not have altered "the social metabolism of capital" (Sen, 2001). But as these alternative ways showed, it can create some spaces for the poor to thwart massive marketization of their lives. But when it concerns health and health services, it should have led to better health and enhanced availability and accessibility of health services. As discussed, the multitudes of decentralization that are presented through a number of channels, frameworks, and institutions have not led to any considerable increase in the degree of autonomy at the lower levels although it could have resulted in increased transparency with respect to allocation and expenditure, enhanced awareness regarding power possibilities and much more visible spread of welfare programs. It is now admitted that decentralization implemented as a reform measure does not guarantee improved efficiency in the delivery of health care or better autonomy in decision-making or better health outcomes. "Numerous conditions, often overlooked, influence the success of decentralization processes, including local managerial and technical capacity, systems of accountability, clear and transparent legal frameworks that delineate the division of responsibilities, and sufficient funding to fulfill mandates and to meet local priorities" (Hutchinson and LaFond, 2004:1).

For the benefits of decentralization or devolution of power to reach the people, and to galvanize the existing channels and opportunities created by political decentralization and concomitantly health sector decentralization in whatever form, an alternate platform needs to be created. This is the subaltern platform of decentralization which could be created by appropriated social mobilization strategies. The negative features of existing decentralization strategies that we identified could be nullified by this within the health service system where the people form the key component and any disorder in that component need to be rectified. These are conditions in addition to those mentioned by Hutchinson and LaFond, overlooked in a bureaucratic framework and the conventional decentralization initiatives.

It is in this context of considering the conditions which preclude people from participating in the process of governance on issues which matter to them, that the issue of marginalization and exclusion need to be seriously grappled. A strategy of focused action is likely to strengthen the existing decentralization initiatives such as "people's planning." There is a need to raise the question regarding the ways to respond to people's needs that are generated from heterogeneity of cultures and diversity of social, economic, and ecological conditions than on appropriateness of systems that distribute economic and political power among various levels of government (Mathur, 1998). Given the extreme vulnerability, exclusion, and discrimination of the poor (CSDH, 2008), and the poor health outcomes among the poor and vulnerable sections, there is a need to undertake specific focused actions with a view to facilitate access to health care, encourage safe deliveries, and child care. Identification of the poor and the vulnerable is a challenging methodological task. As single measures like income or calorie intake are often inaccurate, several indices have been used to identify families below the poverty line. The Kerala State Poverty Eradication Mission known as Kudumbasree uses the following to identify the poor (Government of Kerala, 2002). Families with four or more of the factors below are listed as poor and vulnerable.

- No land / less than 10 cents of land
- No house/dilapidated house
- No sanitary latrine
- No access to safe drinking water within 300 meters
- Women headed household / presence of a widow, divorcee / abandoned lady / unwed mother
- No regularly employed person in the family
- Socially disadvantaged groups (SC/ST)
- Presence of mentally or physically challenged person / chronically ill member in the family
- Families with an illiterate adult member

Having identified the poor and vulnerable, from a pragmatic and practical point of view it is important to identify the pathways in order to initiate health care strategies which can have epidemiological effectiveness and ensure people's participation. Embodiment is a necessary element for piloting such pathways. Embodiment in this case means generating evidence regarding the processes that lead to morbidity or mortality which needs a holistic and epidemiological vision. This vision has to be docked with the political face of health programs. Obviously, this requires a multidimensional approach and many of our current evidences regarding the relationships between body, ill-health, and social factors including poverty do not adopt such multidimensional and multi-level approach. The evidences are often dichotomized as upstream and downstream or distal and proximal factors and in that process marginalize the more difficult to attain upstream or distal factors. Let us consider maternal and child health (MCH) as an illustration.

Formation of Empowered Action Groups of Women in Villages

If we consider maternal and child health (MCH) which is one of the most priority problems identified in health policies and international policies such as Millennium Development Goals, an action-oriented model can be evolved (Nayar, 2011). Given the cultural and social norms attached to pregnancy, child birth, and child rearing, the best possible pathway for the health programs is through the women themselves. The village-level health services should be able to form an Empowered Action Group (EAG) of women who can guide the program for the focused actions. The composition of the group should be based on age, social background, leadership qualities etc. In other words, this deliberative action could form the democratic component of the program through which ideals of primary health care can be realized in this third decade of the Alma Ata declaration. Such committees with multidimensional tasks can strive to achieve convergence between health programs and other social sector programs.

Multi-level Social Sector Actions on Maternal and Child Mortality

Based on the available evidence regarding social determinants leading to poor maternal and child health outcomes, we propose the following model which

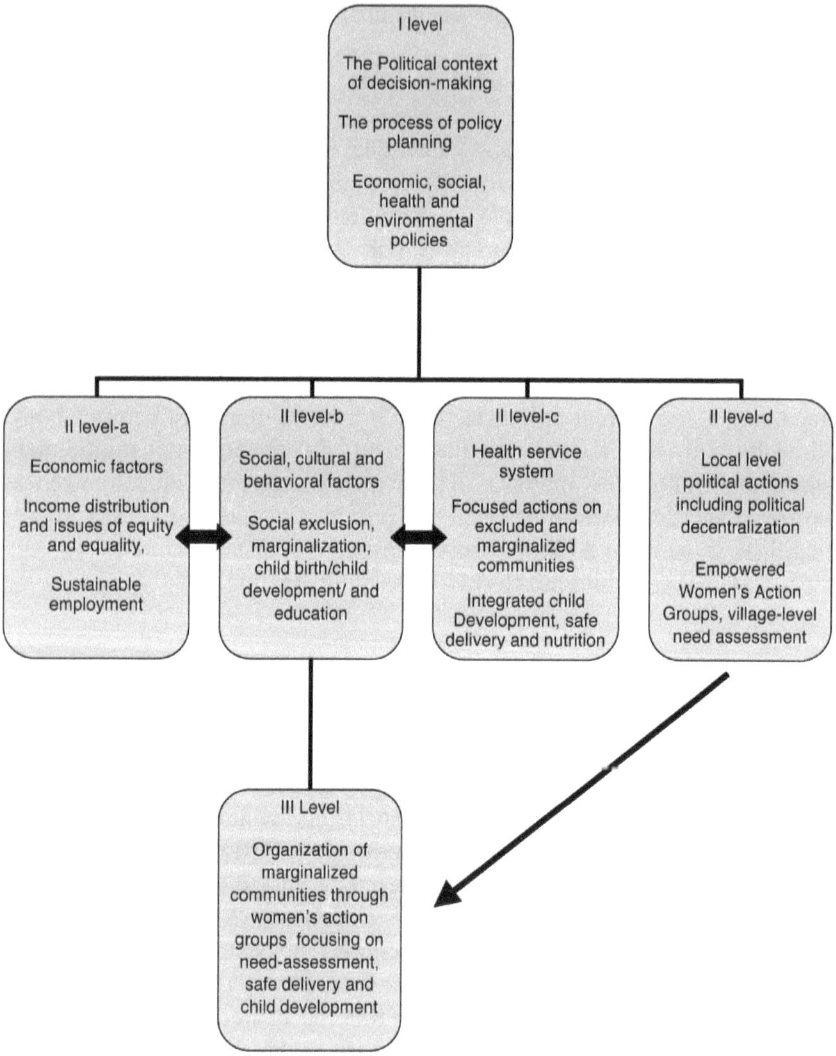

Figure 4.1. Decentralization for universal maternal and child health: An alternative model

is a set of mainly three pragmatic actions which can be undertaken synergistically. Some of these actions especially the *process of policy-making* (I level) and *economic factors such as employment generation* (II level a) require actions at the political level.

A number of convergent and intersectoral actions can be undertaken jointly by health services and other sectors at the micro-level. These are measures which evolve as a corollary to the discussions in the previous sections and to address some of the problems identified therein. It is evident that such an intersectoral action will be "strongest, and outcomes are best, when the collaboration is both vertical and horizontal . . . weaving these elements together yields a resilient and durable end product, and provides a shield against inaction, flagging interest, or disintegration" (WHO and PHAC, 2008).

The II level includes all the factors which could be identified at the micro-level. The actions proposed, to be initiated at the micro level, are:

- Organization of marginalized groups in the villages (focused group actions) to address the problem of social exclusion and to ensure equal opportunity by affirmative action.
- Formation of empowered action groups of women (given the close linkage between education, empowerment, and health) who could influence fellow women which could help in moving toward a safe and vibrant MNCH program.
- Given the paucity of data, a decentralized data gathering mechanism can be evolved through the channels mentioned above. This data can also be used for enhancing epidemiological efficiency of the program and as a need-assessment strategy.

Such a multilevel and multidimensional approach to decentralization could add to the vibrancy of the existing institutionally driven programs and help to achieve some degree of sustainability through public participation. The role of civil society is closely intertwined with these initiatives and the dynamics of their role is dissected in the next chapter.

5

Civilizing the Civil Society and Civilians

Old Bottles and New Medicines

Civil society is not just an ephemeral fad created by the international developmental agencies but the concept has also evolved out of scholastic inputs and has been sharpened by plethora of academic debates and discussions in the knowledge kilns of western sociology and political science. Among the scholars, Thomas Hobbes, John Locke, Montesquieu, Hegel, Marx, and more importantly Gramsci have been responsible for the conceptual shifts after considerable chiseling. The dialectical relationships between the state and the civil society and the conceptualization of civil society as one institution with shared values, ideas, and meanings as pointed out by Gramsci seem to have influenced much of the theoretical debates. However, similar to decentralization, even after such eminent treatments of the term, the confusions regarding the term civil society are rampant but they are discussed in detail by many other scholars and we will only give a passing reference to these discourses (Nayar, 2005). It is now accepted that the term, based on its ideological underpinnings, has a number of strands. Without getting entangled in the theoretical strands which have been eloquently discussed by Kaviraj, one can easily surmise based on his discussions that there is a "conceptual unclarity" with the term and it is necessary to understand the undifferentiated variety of states and civil societies in the South and probably undifferentiated so-called federal states within the state (Kaviraj, 2001). It is also unclear as to how the non-state actors are identified or classified. Obviously, those who had a blind faith on the instrumental utilitarian approach did not bother too much with these eloquent theoretical probematique for operationalizing their ideological predilections. The disjunction with the scholarly inputs and the practical applications is quite evident.

CIVIL SOCIETY IN HEALTH

Two important landmarks in the 20th century—the emergence of large number of postcolonial states and much later the collapse of the Soviet Union and the emergence of a large number of former socialist countries—could have led to a renewed interest in the civil society. In both situations, the issue of a weak state with poor resources was pointed out as a handicap for ensuring a dignified life for its citizens. The continued existence of sub-human conditions including ill-health in some countries especially sub-Saharan Africa led to the international policy forums to search for appropriate strategic actions to ameliorate the conditions. Thus there emerged the renewed attention on non-state actors for developmental work especially by the aid agencies which mistrusted the state channels. Civil society has in recent times become central in India due to a series of collaborations as well as confrontations in the field of employment, food security, as well as corruption, to name of a few. Although apparently, the state had heeded to these pressures, the outcomes of these positive measures could have been less outstanding.

The international development and aid agencies, in the name enhancing efficiency, have found the constituents of civil society—private enterprises, church and faith-based organizations, co-operatives, NGOs—convenient platforms to by-pass and in the course deemphasize the state (Khilnani, 2001). "To all who invoke it, civil society incarnates a desire to recover for society powers—economic, social, expressive—believed to have been illegitimately usurped by states" (Ibid.:12). The engagement with civil society is also seen in extremely idealistic sense which brands it as the legitimate public actor or as the most effective way to create a healthy and sustainable public life (Naidoo and Tandon, 1999). It is also conceived as the vehicle to infuse life and meaning into democratic practices. It is another matter that since the nineties, they have largely functioned as vehicles of an agenda preset in the funding strategies of international developmental aid agencies. In that process, some of these have also become extremely bureaucratized and formalized and operate as power centers. It is well-known that civil society space and action was not always emancipatory and it was also a site for conflicts and that the sphere of action could be captured by the elites to serve their interests (Tandon and Mohanty, 2002).

With respect to public health, it has become an important component of the discourse and action in recent times again due to the preponderance of the reform model which purported to enhance the efficiency of the government by de-concentration and delegation. It is indeed startling that with a meagre 3–4 percent of the GDP of international health funding, the multi-lateral and bi-lateral funding agencies could wrestle their way into the health programs of developing countries. Such an ideological invasion could be observed in newly independent states carved out of the former Soviet Union and former socialist states and even in newly created states in India such as Jharkhand, Uttarakhand and Chattisgarh.

In the health sector in India, the role of civil society in the form of a pressure group since the nineties has been less promising as compared to for instance, the anti-corruption or food security movements despite the presence of organizations such as people's health movement or *Jan Swasthya Abhiyan* and Medico Friends Circle. Historically, however, there were recommendations emanating from many health committees set-up by the Indian National Congress and the government of India suggesting the active participation of civil society in health programs.

The Sokhey committee suggested utilizing existing *akharas* (wrestling training schools), educational or social clubs or religious societies (of all faiths and creeds) for active cooperation to form a rural health service (National Planning Committee, 1948). It also suggested that health advisory committees should be formed composed of leading citizens (Ibid.:71–72). It mentions that festivals such as diwali, Id, holi etc. could be used to spread health awareness. The report hoped that many evils of the country may be removed and corrupted religious practices reformed with the approval of religious leaders and reformers! (Ibid.:73)

The Bhore committee had also been vocal about involving the civil society and especially it had specific recommendations for enhancing people's participation by setting up health committees (Government of India, 1946). It also suggested the importance of involving voluntary organizations in anti-Tuberculosis activities. For rural housing, the committee suggested forming neighborhood units for planning various utilities associated with living in a rural area (Ibid., Vol. 3: 88). Basically, the committee was concerned about how a health program can be operationalized and made effective given the social and economic conditions of the people. By using words such as apathy, lack of consciousness and awareness, the report suggests ways to enlist the support of the people. For instance with regard to environmental sanitation, the committee says, "This lack of regard for community hygiene can be remedied only by an awakening of a health consciousness among the people. Experience shows that, in the absence of such awakening, improvement in the sanitation of the environment is difficult and often impossible even with the provision of appropriate public services" (Ibid., Vol. 2: 45). According to the committee, "a spirit of self-help should be created among the people through the development of co-operative effort for the purpose of promoting curative and preventive health work. In the program of health development, which we put forward, the need for securing the active cooperation of the people in the day to day functioning of the health organization should be prominently kept in view (Ibid., Vol. 1:19). The committee thought that "the vast majority of the people of India view with apathy the large amount of unnecessary suffering and morbidity that exists in their midst and, unless this attitude can be replaced by one of active cooperation among themselves an. with the health authorities for the promotion of the health of the community, no permanent success can be achieved. The most effective way of helping to create such a change in outlook is, we believe by providing for the people opportunities of active participation in the local health program" (Ibid., Vol. 2:44).

Against this background, the committee visualized forming health committees in all the villages given the existence of *panchayats* in the villages. To again quote from the report, "the principle of the *panchayat* or a council of five elders who, through their collective wisdom, direct community life in the village has long been applied in practice in India. We desire to see local health committees set up on this principle of bringing together certain number of persons of standing in the village who can be helpful in promoting specific lines of health activity. In selecting such persons we do not wish to bring in the vote and the spirit of competition for the vote which however desirable it may be for conferring on these individuals the right of claiming to be representative of the people, has also the disadvantage of introducing into the peaceful atmosphere of cooperative effort, which we are proposing to create, the heat and controversy of the political arena. At the same time there should be a large measure of popular support for these individuals" (Ibid., Vol. 2:44–45).

The Health Survey and Planning Committee in 1962, popularly known as the Mudaliar committee, also considered a memorandum on health cooperatives. This is indeed surprising given the thrust of the committee on strengthening and consolidating existing government health services in the country (Government of India, 1962).[1] The Bajaj committee much later mentions community resources, people and their participation as vital for the success health programs (Government of India, 1987).

> The essence and essential of Primary Health Care is community participation. Without the active participation of people in the management of their own health care, it will be impossible to raise the status and standard of health. As such, the community itself becomes a major resource in developing effective and efficient health service in the country. For this a massive effort towards community mobilization for health will have to be mounted. Community awareness, community sensitization, and community action constitute the essential pre-requisites for a well-planned program of action aimed at mobilization of community resources. (Ibid:12)

The foregoing historical snapshot shows that "people" and "civil society" were required to facilitate the spread of health services and therefore, the role was purely instrumental. Given this historical context, I will examine the three faces of civil society—the public benefit organizations such as NGOs and mutual benefit organizations such as co-operatives and self help groups—which have been heralded as important "stakeholders" for extending and facilitating health services to the people.

NGOS IN HEALTH CARE

This is the most tried-out option outside the state largely due to the ideological push by the funding agencies. Voluntary, non-profit and non-governmental actions have become part of the same universe of the so-called Third sector organizations (TSOs) although distinctions are important in terms of formality, professionalism, interests, organization, etc. (Lewis, 1999; Sarkar, 2005). Such third-sector actions, as mentioned earlier, are co-terminus with the emergence of structural adjustment/reform agenda and alternative visions of political systems beyond the dichotomies of capitalism and socialism with the end of Soviet Union and the emergence of a large number of newly independent countries and political entities within countries. Such adjustment or reform agenda has led to calls for "less government" and "reinventing government" (Chuengsatiansup, 2008). These two options are ideologically tilted toward the reform process while critics of reforms argue for strengthening the government and the public sector (Qadeer, Sen, and Nayar, 2001). Theoretical work examining the role of networks and affiliations on shaping societal structures including concepts such as social capital and more concrete instrumental processes such as communitization have also contributed to the immense interest in non-state actors. The communitization drive under the NRHM has initiated a number of programs such as village health and sanitation committee, village health and nutrition days, space for public participation in hospital development committees and in district health societies and the support to community monitoring programs. Micro studies have also shown that the involvement of non-state actors such as voluntary workers and community leaders can substantially help in improving service delivery such as immunization (Das et. al, 2000).

Service delivery is the main focus of activity among NGOs in developing countries under a donor-driven agenda privatization agenda (Edwards, 1999). As discussed by Edwards, this is similar to the trend in industrialized countries in the 1980s when widespread privatization of the welfare state happened under rhetoric of public-private partnership. The performance of such service deliveries are also measured according to market and managerial values. "In cases like Bangladesh a focus on service delivery is understandable given widespread state and market failure, the size of gaps in the provision of even the most basic of services, anti-NGO sentiments among religious groups, journalists and others, deeply-entrenched social and political elites and a government which is wary of any other form of NGO activity" (Ibid.: 261). The Indian context was not as grave as the above scenario and the gaps and failures were to some extent synthetic and not real. The ideology of non-state action was constructed on an image of apparently dysfunctional state under the neo-liberal reforms.

The NGO has become an integral component of "Indian social landscape" and its contribution to economic development and social change is discussed widely (Beteille, 2005). What have become prominent in the health sector among various third sector organizations are the NGOs largely due to the neo-liberal agenda engulfing the social sectors. Non-governance of the health administration was to some extent responsible for the acceptance of the third sector. Their role in health care also became widespread in the late eighties when a number of international organizations entered the field of health care funding for different health programs, HIV/ADS being the most prominent. State was often characterized as inefficient and considered ill equipped to handle issues such as health. This inefficiency argument was applied to both issues of financing as well as the implementation of health programs. The NGOs were considered as a viable option as they fall between completely state-oriented services and privatized care.

NGOs are normally outside direct state control, non-profit-making with a voluntary decision-making structure and a partially formalized organization (Green and Matthias, 1997: 25). There are broadly two categories of NGOs, single-country (CYNGOs) and international (INGOs). However, there are various combinations of NGOs at different levels, the community-based NGOs, which are regional or local and which operate at the sub-national level and the National NGOs, which operate at the country level. Health NGOs are involved in a number of activities such as service provision, implementation targeted programs, research and project preparation including consultancy, policy advocacy, etc. Rough estimates show that there are about 80,000 development NGOs which also work on health issues and if registration under appropriate state legislations are considered, then the number reduces to around 32,000 as in 2006 (Kilby, 2011). The main driving force of NGOs apart from donor-defined programs and funds is the value of service provision for public interest. The vibrant history of NGOs in India shows that they have evolved into a broad-based sector but still riddled with problems of autonomy and independence (Ibid.:18). We are also witnessing reducing role of state-control on NGOs but they are kept away from political processes and mainly as empowering agencies with a few exceptions in recent times.

It appears that although the golden period of NGOs is getting over, the international and national policy documents still favor their role in some aspects of health. The attitude toward NGOs is shifting from dogmatic rejection or acceptance to a more realistic and useful pragmatism (Green and Matthias, 1997). However, there is no firm evidence that NGOs have an advantage over State, although they may be useful in some sectors like relief operations etc. under certain conditions (Green and Matthias:59–60). There is now a willingness to be critical of the role of NGOs in the health sector especially considering cases from Bangladesh where paradoxes and dilemmas were discernible and Mozambique where inefficiency and lack of sensitivity have crept into the operation of NGOs (Green and Matthias:45). A number of recent impact studies have shown that with regard to criteria such as reaching the poorest, coverage, cost-effectiveness, quality of services, or policy direction, non-governmental development organizations do not have any advantage over the State (UNRISD: 95). As concentration of funding and projects increase, "NGOs become susceptible to bureaucratisation, self-aggrandizement, and imposition of standardized solutions" (Wolfe, 1994:20). In such a context, "the claim that NGO projects are more innovative and staff more dedicated and responsive to local circumstances then becomes less likely to be true" (Ibid.:20). However, it is doubtful whether the bubble of NGOs will burst in the early periods of this millennium. There could be a reduction in their role probably due to the increased activities of the private sector. As is evident from the literature, there is some degree of ambiguity regarding the role of NGOs in health care largely due to the diversity of NGOs, the range of activities and the countries they are operating, etc. (Green and Matthias, 1997). This ambiguity regarding the advantage of NGOs has resulted in their continuing support by international organizations and national governments. Between 1982 and 1990, there was a steep increase in the external assistance provided to the health sector through the NGOs. It was estimated that although total external assistance to the health sector in 1990 was only US$ 480 million, or only 2.9 percent of total health expenditures in developing countries, 23 percent of this external assistance was provided through NGOs in 1990 (Michaud and Murray, 1994). Reviews undertaken by the WHO also unconditionally support the involvement of civil society organizations on contractual or partnership basis for improving health system performance especially in areas where they complement government functions (Alliance for Health Policy and Systems Research, 2004).

The government of India has been encouraging NGOs to set-up new hospitals and dispensaries in rural areas to improve the existing hospital services

(Government of India, 2002f; Government of India, 2002g). In addition, voluntary organizations running hospitals in rural areas or urban areas are eligible to get financial assistance for expansion and improvement of facilities. In 1999–2000, an outlay of about 17 million rupees had been earmarked in the budget for this purpose. The government has also been giving liberal assistance to NGOs for family planning and RCH programs. For RCH program, NGOs have been classified into three types:

1. Small service NGOs at the village, *panchayat*, and block level for advocacy of RCH and family planning practices and for counseling.
2. Mother NGOs with substantial resources and competence for every 8 to 10 districts with representatives of the state and central governments on its executive committee.
3. The national NGOs, which are to be entrusted work for developing innovative programs.

These NGOs will be involved for specific areas such as introduction of baby friendly practices in hospitals, enforcement of pre-natal diagnostic techniques, act by detecting offending sex determination clinics, etc. Some of these NGOs will also be involved in assisting hospitals in urban areas for offering contraceptive methods and counseling services in RCH and family planning.

The government had also floated the sterilization bed scheme for voluntary organizations way back in 1964. Sterilization bed scheme is a government of India scheme, which encouraged voluntary organizations/NGOS engaged in family welfare activities to participate in National Family Welfare Program by way of ensuring reserved beds available with them for Sterilization purposes. This enabled them to provide facilities for tubectomy operations. Under the scheme, performance-based bed maintenance grant of Rs. 6,000 per bed per annum is provided to the institution on achieving a minimum of 60 tubectomies per bed per annum.

The draft health policy of India (Government of India, 2002h) is another example of this support, perhaps on an expanded scale. It envisaged the role of NGOs in disease control programs. The policy also suggested, considering what it called the high "motivational skills" of these organizations and the significant contribution made by NGOs and other organizations in the civil society that a definite portion of the budget in respect of identified program components should be earmarked for exclusive implementation by NGOs.

This shows that the halo of NGOs still lingers on although in recent times, the initial enthusiasm has declined and there is a realization that ". . . civil society response has been slow in being able to respond on scale. High quality civil society organizations with capacity to deliver and be accountable continue to be few and scattered" (Government of India, 2010:40). One could argue, given the mixed signals emanating from a number of countries regarding the advantage of NGOs, that it is time to question the unbridled faith in such organizations.

CO-OPERATIVES IN HEALTH CARE

Co-operatives are seen as a potential "third realm," and there appears to be a global revival of co-operatives in the social and health fields (United Nations, 2001). As evident from the UN review, co-operatives have been highly successful in the credit sector and in agricultural marketing. Based on such experiences, there is much enthusiasm about the potential of co-operatives in health care provision, and an idealized picture is relayed. However, even proponents have noticed the paucity of studies evaluating the potential of co-operatives for poverty alleviation and the provision of health services (United Nations, 1997; Sinats, 2001). Issues such as the viability of co-operatives in a hierarchical society and the reasons for the decline of co-operatives in the social sector of some developing countries need to be examined before propagating their revival (Nayar and Razum, 2006). This section analyzes the experience from developing countries, in particular China and the states of Gujarat and Kerala, India, to explore the viability of co-operatives as a "third option" for the provision of health care in India as a whole.

Originally started as a consumer organization by impoverished weavers during industrial revolution in England, co-operatives soon evolved into a tool to unleash productive forces. The primary aim of the co-operative, as assumed by many scholars, is to contribute to the welfare of the members by a self-help or mutual-aid process (Selden, 1998). It is also visualized as an open and autonomous organization based on voluntary participation that embodies principles of democratic management.

In the health field, user- and provider-owned co-operatives need to be distinguished. User-owned health co-operatives are set up by community members to help them meet their own health care needs. An equally important aspect is empowerment, as users determine the goals and practices of the health services provided. Co-operative members provide shares of capital and subsequently pay premiums to help cover operating costs. Often, co-operatives negotiate contracts with health insurance and health care providers, or they operate their own services and hospitals (International Co-operative Information Centre, undated). Provider-owned co-operatives are usually formed by doctors who wish to offer a wider range of services, or to contain costs by bulk purchasing and by sharing administrative and technical services (Nayar and Razum, 2006).

A United Nations Global Survey on co-operative enterprises in the health and social care sectors found that co-operative health services operate in more than 50 developed and developing countries, representing or serving around 100 million households around the world. The survey identified three main types of co-operatives, based on their commitment to health and social care (United Nations, 1997):

1. Co-operative enterprises whose business goals are solely concerned with health and social care;
2. Co-operative enterprises whose business goals include, but are not limited to, the health and social care sectors; and
3. Co-operative enterprises whose business goals do not include health and social care but might include the provision of operational support to health and social care co-operatives.

We will focus mainly on user-owned health co-operatives of the first two types.

HEALTH CO-OPERATIVES IN DEVELOPING COUNTRIES

Health co-operatives, especially of the first type, exist in several developing countries such as Bolivia, Brazil, India, Panama, the Philippines, South Africa, Sri Lanka, and Tanzania. For example, USIMED, a user-owned health co-operative in Brazil, provides extensive coverage to the population and is complemented by UNIMED, a provider-owned co-operative of about 73,000 doctors. In Sri Lanka and India, the government financially supports co-operatives, which provide services to middle and lower income households (United Nations, 1997:16–17). Of particular interest are the Chinese experience with co-operative medical services and the experience of hospital co-operatives in Kerala. We will examine them in more detail in the following sections and then draw lessons for the future of health co-operatives in India.

Co-operatives in China

Co-operatives became very successful in socialist China. One example is the experiment with collectives and co-operatives in the pre–1980 period. The post–1980s then witnessed dramatic changes in the structure of co-operatives in the country. The collectives transformed into enterprises in villages and towns (TVEs). These new enterprises work more like profit-oriented private agencies, and workers do not enjoy the same autonomy as in collectives.

Workers who once had guaranteed jobs and enjoyed free or subsidized health care now face lay-offs, have little security and are paid piece rates. In addition, most enterprises are concentrated in the richer coastal suburban areas and in prosperous model villages. Poor regions, particularly those lacking essential infrastructure, have few of these enterprises or other than agricultural co-operatives (Selden, 1988).

The Co-operative Medical Services (CMS) in China were developed along with the collectives in the 1960s and 1970s to ensure access to basic health care for the rural population. The original function of the CMS was to collect voluntary contributions from brigades, production teams and households, to reimburse medical expenses to households and to recruit, train, and monitor barefoot doctors (Xiao-ming et al., 1993; Carrin et al., 1999). The coverage rate of the CMS in rural areas increased consistently until the end of the 1970s when it was estimated to be 90 percent (Liu, Cao, 1992). With the market-oriented economic reforms of the 1980s, production systems shifted from the community to the households, which resulted in the discontinuation of the collective financing of health care. The emphasis of health care has since shifted from lower to higher levels, from preventive to curative services, and from planning and management to market forces (Feng et al., 1995). As a result of reforms, most CMS stations have been closed. In some places, CMS stations have evolved into various other types of medical and health care services; in other places, they ceased to operate altogether. Participation declined from 90 percent of the villages to 10 percent. Health status, as measured by infant mortality rate and incidence of infectious diseases has worsened in areas where CMS have ceased to operate (Zhu et al., 1989). Villagers' expenditure on health care has increased. In the absence of CMS, the rural population has to pay for health care out-of-pocket, and poor families have greater difficulty in getting access to basic health care (Xing-Yuan, Sheng-Lan, 1995; Liu, Wang, 1991).

Reasons for the Decline of CMS

The major reason for the decline of CMS in China was the change in the financing system and the resulting lack of incentive for the individuals to participate. There was no cash withholding system and no efficient channel to collect health and welfare funds for CMS operations. By relying on voluntary contributions from households instead of mandatory contribution, it was not possible to sustain CMS funding. Apart from this, mixed signals from the leadership changed the attitude toward CMS in the rural areas (Xiao-ming et al., 1993). Many local administrators perceived that the CMS no longer enjoyed the backing of the central government. This shows that co-operatives in China, although based on the principle of collectivism, have functioned largely as para-state organizations.

Revival of CMS

There still exists in China a positive attitude toward collective medical and health organization, as large sections of the rural population do not have coverage for curative services (Xiao-ming et al., 1993). Attempts are being made to revive the CMS and community financing in some counties. The revival of CMS however is not based on the principles of collectivism that prevailed earlier. Even those CMS, which continued to exist after the widespread collapse were kept intact only because of a local capacity to provide funds. Thus they survived only in the rich areas similar to the TVEs. The new generation of rural co-operative health care schemes has evolved into a medical insurance system under the guidance of health administrators and insurance companies. The current thinking on the reestablishment of CMS is thus influenced by the basic principles of insurance. The focus is on village-based schemes, with minimal external funding and no reimbursement of drug costs and payments for secondary and tertiary care (Hao et al., 1998). The experience of a pilot project in 14 counties has not been very encouraging although there were instances of modest reduction in the cost of health care on families in some counties (Carrin et al., 1999: 972). The revived CMS could also lead to a shift from preventive to curative medicine and higher expenditure for tertiary care. (Bogg et al., 1996). It is doubtful whether this experiment can consolidate the three-tier network of health services consisting of countryside doctors, village health centers, and county hospitals. The evidence currently available indicates that a re-establishment of CMS cannot overcome the problem of low access for the poorer households unless there are specific and effective mechanisms to finance their inclusion, and willingness of higher levels of governments to subsidise the services (Hao et al., 1998; Yunguo, Bloom, 2002). More governmental promotion and support and funds from multiple sources would be required for the reestablishment of CMS (Liu et al.,1996). As the insurance philosophy dominates the running of the program, it would become more and more inaccessible to the poorer sections.

The Experience from Gujarat and Kerala

The Indian experience with co-operatives is more diverse than that of China, although to a large extent co-operatives in India also functioned as an appendage of the state. In most states of India, co-operatives are the primary testing ground for local level electoral politics. Most co-operatives were planned without adequate knowledge about the life of the villagers and were based on a so-called "blueprint approach" (Hyden, 1988), which means that their design followed a universal mold rather than local requirements. The co-operative sector is largely considered as an instrument of production or as an agency which would facilitate production. Therefore, we find credit and marketing co-operatives in sectors such as milk, sugar, tea, agriculture, fertilizers, fisheries, handloom weaving, etc., and very few in the social sectors. One of the earliest evaluation studies revealed that the factors behind successful co-operatives are their favorable location, good communication facilities besides the presence of a vigorous co-operatives movement and a helpful central financial agency (Government of India, 1960:121). Co-operatives, whether formal or informal, whether based on grass roots or state planning, are not likely to change the indigenous social structure very much as they do not reach all segments of society equally (Attwood and Baviskar, 1988). There is considerable evidence now showing that co-operatives do not provide equal opportunities to different socio-economic groups; in this respect, rural areas and especially the poorest members of society are at a disadvantage (George, 1994).

Emergence of Health Co-operatives

The experience with health co-operatives in India is not very extensive. A health co-operative movement of a limited scale had existed in the 1920s and 1930s in Bengal, Madras, and the Punjab (United Nations, 1997:15–16). Curative and preventive health activities as well as mother-and-child care were the activities of the user-owned, community-based health co-operatives established in the Birbhum District of Bengal. In the Punjab and the United Province, the activities of the *better-living co-operative societies* were broadly similar to health co-operatives. However, there was no continuity between the pre– and post–World War movements. Most of the postwar health-oriented co-operatives were established in the western and southern states of Maharastra, Goa, Karnataka and Kerala. The Mudaliar committee sponsored a report on medical care programs in India which covered health cooperatives as well. The report was based on a study tour in India in 1958 by Ralph G. Victor, an American co-operator (Victor, 1962). The main purpose of this report was to examine the possibility of evolving self-supported medical care programs in India. After analyzing several medical plans including many co-operatives, the report concluded that there is little likelihood of consumer-controlled, pre-payment medical co-operatives, run without government support, will succeed in India. However, the report gave several reasons in support of establishing medical co-operatives. The foremost was the focus on democratization of health care which would enable each citizen to develop as an individual according to his needs and abilities and enhance participation of people in the social, political, and economic institutions surrounding him (Ibid.:53). Other reasons included:

1. Government cannot provide the level of medical care people want
2. Most people cannot afford private care
3. It may help in better distribution of doctors away from cities (Ibid.:54).

Health-oriented Co-operatives—The SEWA Initiative

In the postwar period, co-operative movements associated with the informal/NGO sector have achieved some degree of success although their goals are not limited to health. The *Self-Employed Women's Association* (SEWA) of Ahemedabad in the Gujarat state used the co-operative and self-help approach to organise the workers in the non-organised sectors. The SEWA has an extensive and complex organisational structure with an apex union, co-operatives and support services (Jhabvala and Bali, undated). It comprises about 85 co-operatives, mostly involved in production-oriented activities (SEWA, 2000). Women workers provide the share capital and obtain employment in the co-operatives. One woman can become member of one or more co-operative. A democratically elected executive committee of workers runs the co-operatives.

SEWA has set-up training schools for health workers and midwives. Staffs trained by these schools carry out health activities in nine districts of the state. Health workers and midwives have also formed co-operatives with the aim of improving the health of women workers (SEWA, 2000). Within its multi-purpose and multi-faceted approach, SEWA provides community-based integrated primary health care, referral services, health education, cataract operations, immunisation, as well as case-finding and treatment for TB (Bhatt, 1996). However, initially complete coverage of the members could not been achieved even with the extensive organisational structure (Jhabvala, undated:50).

Medical Co-operatives in Kerala

Kerala was one of the very few states in India where medical co-operatives were set up in large numbers under government patronage; they have not been studied as extensively as the Chinese CMS, however (Nayar, 2000). The medical co-operatives in Kerala developed during the early 1970s in the aftermath of the Indo-Pakistan war. The war was followed by an acute economic recession, which, in turn, resulted in a severe funding crisis in the social sectors and rising unemployment among graduates from the government-owned medical colleges in the state. About 450 villages in Kerala were medically underserved, and co-operatives were considered as a viable alternative approach for providing basic medical care to the people, and, at the same time, for accommodating the new medical graduates (Government of Kerala, 1998). The focus of these co-operatives was limited to medical care instead of comprehensive health care. Issues such as equitable access to medical care and the political and social dimensions of co-operatives were not addressed at the time. Although there was some social purpose in this initiative, it was primarily an *ad hoc* stopgap for providing employment to the medical graduates. Based on the experience during the initial years, co-operative rural dispensaries as self-contained medical units were established in the late seventies in several districts with the idea of containing government expenditure for social sectors (George, 1976). These dispensaries were expected to supplement the work of the primary health centers and government dispensaries at a lesser cost to the public exchequer.

At present, many of these co-operative institutions, especially the dispensaries in the rural areas, are either not functioning or functioning sub-optimally (see table 5.1).

The proportion of institutions incurring losses has been increasing, and it can be observed that around 65 percent of the institutions had become non-profitable by 1993–94, although membership had increased substantially.

Reasons for the Decline of the Medical Co-operatives

The decline of the medical co-operatives in Kerala started in the 1980s after the coverage of the public sector health services had considerably expanded (Panikkar and Soman, 1984). By that time, at least one government dispensary with a doctor was in place in most of the villages and some form of curative care was available in the villages. With improved accessibility of

Table 5.1. Profile of medical co-operatives in Kerala

	1973–74	*1983–84*	*1993–94*
Number of co-operatives	64	72	137
Members	17 976	19 930	59 066
Profitable	6 (9.4%)	14 (19.4%)	19 (13.9%)
Non-profitable	—	31 (43.1%)	89 (65.0%)
No loss, no profit	—	27 (37.5%)	29 (21.1%)

Source: Nayar, 2000

public sector health services, the interest of the state in medical co-operatives gradually declined. Furthermore, the private sector grew significantly during subsequent years (Thankappan, 2001), setting up a parallel, profit-oriented system of health services that competed with the medical co-operatives. The third sector health services could not compete with the reasonably and fairly distributed public sector health care and the readily available.

Increasing competition exposed the most important reasons for the failure of medical co-operatives in Kerala, namely inadequate managerial and technical inputs (Government of Kerala, 1998). For example, out of the ninety-two dispensaries, eighty-two are functioning sub-optimally due to a lack of working capital and of committed staff, including doctors (ibid.). Employees perceive service conditions as unsatisfactory because of lacking incentives, career paths and resources. Most of the co-operatives did not have any autonomy in decision-making with respect to its day-to-day functioning, and there was over-politicisation and centralisation of power in a few individuals (Nambiar, 1996). Doctors and other technical staff were underrepresented on the governing body of the co-operatives.

Structural problems confound the situation; membership of the co-operations is limited, there are no incentives for the institution such as special tax concessions or building assistance etc., and patients are not channelled to the appropriate level of care as there is no three-tier system divided into primary, central, and apex institutions (Government of Kerala, 1998). Ultimately, only those co-operative institutions, especially the hospitals that were managed like private enterprises could survive. Out of the fifty-seven co-operative hospitals, thirty-three are functioning at an optimal level. These co-operative hospitals are profit-oriented; they have sufficiently large catchment areas, and can afford high-tech diagnostic and therapeutic facilities. To a certain extent, they can even moderate the exploitative practices of the private hospitals (Nambiar, 1996).

Increasingly, there is a trend in developing countries to introduce market-oriented strategies in the state hospitals as a part of health sector reforms and to create economically autonomous hospitals (Hanson et al., 2001). In India, several state governments have embarked on strategies to privatise public hospitals and even primary care institutions (Bhat, 2000). The undesirable consequences such as rising costs, increasing inequity, and consumer exploitation (Purohit, 2001) are not often addressed in public-private partnership (PPP) strategies. Are medical co-operatives a viable solution in the present context of public health crisis in India? There is no broad evidence base so far indicating that co-operatives can provide comprehensive curative and preventive health services in the same way as the public sector health services. The experience with the Chinese model of co-operatives prior to the reform period provides evidence that they could achieve universal coverage of basic health services. On the other hand, medical co-operatives failed in Kerala as an alternative due to a strong public sector health service. Co-operatives can probably play a complimentary role in the transition from governmental to a private health care provision but they require strong government support to be viable. NGO-sponsored co-operatives (type 1 in table 5.2), which provide preventive and some minimum curative support, do not need much external input and could serve as models for evolving primary care units. A mix of type 2 and type 3 co-operatives is suitable for secondary and tertiary services which should then be closely linked to the primary level by a social insurance approach.

Positive outlook regarding health co-operatives emerges from descriptive reports rather than rigorous analytical and empirical studies. A number of relevant issues are so far unresolved or not yet supported by sufficient evidence to inform decision-making in India. Firstly, most experience with the risk-sharing concept in the context of health co-operatives derives from industrialised countries. More experience from developing countries with relatively lower and/or less regular incomes and families with larger number of dependents is needed to establish the minimum number of members for such schemes to be operationally viable. Secondly, there is a need to understand the comparative advantage (cost-effectiveness, user willingness/satisfaction, coverage, accessibility to the poor and disadvantaged sections, etc.) between government health care and co-operatives. Evidence from China shows that

Table 5.2. Comparison of health-related co-operatives in India and China

Types/ Characteristics	*Type 1: NGO sponsored, SEWA (India)*	*Type 2: State sponsored, Kerala (India)*	*Type 3: Collective–Commune, China*
Health orientation	Primary care	Mainly curative	Curative and preventive
Ownership	Run by health workers and women	Considerable government inputs	Government support but resources from the community
Governance	Self-help model	Run as private enterprises	Decentralised governance
Approach	Social insurance approach	Fee-for-service approach	Social insurance approach

Source: Nayar and Razum, 2006

co-operatives tend to become dysfunctional when state support is withdrawn (unlike in developed countries where they are autonomous entities). Hence, the role of co-operatives as an alternative to government health services is questionable. The advantage of fully autonomous co-operatives over state-controlled co-operatives has also not been systematically studied although international policies prescribe autonomous self-sustaining co-operatives for rural development (Hussi et al., 1993).

In India, health co-operatives as a "third option" in health care do not seem viable. They are not a general solution that can be "prescribed" to compensate for deteriorating access to health services following market-oriented health sector reforms, particularly not in view of the increasing demand for clinical care in the coming years and impoverishment of the people (Nayar and Razum, 2006).

SELF-HELP FOR HEALTH CARE AS A THIRD OPTION

The paradigm of health sector reforms currently undertaken at the global level has also influenced the move toward another third sector such as the self-help groups or SHGs. This section discusses the self-help approach as a third option, its pattern and explores its viability in the health sector of developing countries. Many scholars have repeatedly advocated self-help in health care. Recently, for example, micro-finance groups/enterprises have been suggested as an option for community health financing (Perker et al., 2002). Still, there have been no efforts to critically evaluate the relevance of self-help in the present context. The question that needs to be addressed is: Can government health services in developing countries be partially replaced by self-help, thus reducing health care expenditure; or can self-help groups merely complement the social and health services offered (and funded) by a functioning social welfare state? This section is based on published sources, some of which are not directly relevant for health. It provides a definition of self-help groups, depict their historical background, assess scope and limitations of the self-help movement in Europe where it originated, document selected experiences in Bangladesh and India, and draw preliminary conclusions regarding the appropriateness of self-help groups for improving population health in developing countries in general and India in particular.

The Self-help Approach

The desirability of empowering communities to take care of their health problems themselves has been raised since long. Often it is argued that self-help is an ingredient of the primary health care strategy with its focus on "peoples' health in peoples' hands" (Robinson, 1980). The strong point could be its orientation toward action and progress; people would learn to be in the role of health care providers in the process. One of the core principles of self-help is that only those experiencing the problem can understand it (Robinson, 1981). This is reflected in the comprehensive and still up-to-date definition of self-help groups given by Katz and Bender 1976 (cited in Katz, 1981:135-136):

> Self-help groups are voluntary, small group structures for mutual aid and the accomplishment of a special purpose. They are usually formed by peers who have come together for mutual assistance in satisfying a common need, overcoming a common handicap or life-disrupting problem, and bringing about desired social and/or personal change. The initiators and members of such groups perceive that their needs are not, or cannot be, met by or through existing social institutions. Self-help groups emphasize face-to-face social interactions and the assumption of personal responsibility by members. They often provide material assistance, as well as emotional support; they are frequently "cause"-oriented, and promulgate an ideology or values through which members may attain an enhanced sense of personal identity.

Katz highlights that self-help groups typically start from a condition of powerlessness, and that the members spontaneously (i.e., not urged by an outside authority) agree on engaging in some actions in which they personally participate. Self-help groups create, and act within, a purposefully organized setting; this distinguishes them from medical self-care, which is practiced by individuals alone or within a family (Katz, 1981).

Self-help in South Asia

As governments and civil society organizations of developing countries, especially those in South Asia, have taken up the concept of self-help, the agenda has become broader and even more ambitious than in industrialized countries. Not only are self-help groups supposed to provide psycho-social support and information to patients and their relatives (Osborne, 1997; Jayaseelan, 1993) and to perform some limited form of primary health care, they are also expected to improve financial accessibility of health care; to ensure sustainability of social services; and to contribute toward income generation (thus, in effect, transforming and expanding self-help groups into economically oriented co-operatives). A typology of self-help groups in Bangladesh and India is evolved in order to derive some preliminary conclusions on the role of self-help groups within the health system of developing countries relative to the experience in industrialized countries (Nayar, Kyobutungi, and

Razum, 2004). The typology is based on 1) the origin of self-help—whether endogenous or exogenous, 2) the approach followed by the self-help groups vis-à-vis their purpose and targets, 3) the type of activities performed by the self-help groups in health, and 4) the sustainability of the groups.

Self-help under NGO Sponsorship

The 1990s marked the arrival of structural adjustment and economic liberalization in India. Concurrently, the number of self-help groups linked with commercial banks increased from 255 in 1992–1993 to 2700 in 1995 (Franco and Kalpana, 1999). Around 85 percent of these groups were formed exclusively by women in production-oriented and income generation activities such as garment making, food processing, etc., and were following a market-oriented approach with a narrow economic focus. These self-help groups were organized with the help of outside agencies and the support of social, religious or political leadership and were seen as alternatives in rural development to break away from the traditional bureaucracy and top-down management (Rajagopal, 1999). A number of non-governmental organizations started self-help groups mainly as savings and credit groups without any emphasis on health. This was an alternative movement due to the failure or absence of a formal rural credit system (Karmakar, 1999). The Grameen Bank of Bangladesh is one of the earliest such movements. In most of the above cases, women were the target group under an approach to development which advocated micro-enterprises in the context of rolling back of the state, the removal of welfare provision, and dismantling of labor protection (Mayoux, 2001). However, available evidence shows that such an approach has failed to make any significant impact on the incomes of poor women over a sustained period and did not lead to any reduction in the gender inequality (Mayoux, 2001).

The Self-Employed Women's Association (SEWA) in Gujarat, India, is a combination of self-help groups and cooperatives of women workers in the informal sector. It followed a multi faceted empowerment approach, wherein all economic activities of the groups were linked to health and social issues, as against the market-oriented approach (Mayoux, 2001). However, there continue to be intensive material and managerial inputs from the apex association in the organization and maintenance of the groups and co-operatives. SEWA has identified and trained midwives and health workers from among the self-help groups. They serve as health educators-cum-barefoot doctors to all the women members of different groups and help the women's groups in forging linkages with the government and private health care providers for specific services and programs. The activities of these health workers include health promotion and preventive health care through health education, immunization, micro-nutrient supplementation, family planning, provision of rational drugs, low-cost traditional medicine, etc. (SEWA, 2000). Subsequently, these health workers have formed their own co-operatives in a move toward achieving sustainability.

The Mahalir Association for Literacy, Awareness and Rights (MALAR) was established in the Kanyakumari District, Tamil Nadu, India, as a women's savings group with the purpose of mobilizing women belonging to the oppressed strata of the society through a structure independent of the government (Franco and Kalpana, 1999). The MALAR experiment, which followed an empowerment approach, is an entirely self-reliant movement without any external funding, but facilitated by external actors. Like SEWA, it has an organizational structure similar to co-operatives, with self-help groups forming the basis. It is also running a health campaign, apart from trying to expand the activities to a women's library movement, legal aid activities, etc. Several districts in Tamil Nadu, Karnataka, Uttar Pradesh, Assam, and Himachal Pradesh have also started such initiatives.

Leading NGOs in Bangladesh have tried a self-help approach for poverty alleviation by forming organizations of poor women (Mushtaque et al., 2001). The activities, apart from income and employment generation, included conscientization, raising awareness for gender equity, and human resource training. The Bangladesh experience is important given the fact that micro-finance/credit and income generation experiments in South Asia started in that country.

A conference organized jointly by three Red Cross Societies, UNDP, and a number of other organizations revealed the renewed interest in self-help, viewing it as a cost-effective and sustainable approach to social development, especially health (Self-help Promotion Secretariat, 2001). The papers presented were based on the experience of about 40 NGOs working in Bangladesh. The NGOs considered the self-help approach largely as a tool for community management. Of special significance was that among the multitude of NGOs working in different sectors of the country, some reported facing problems in phasing-out their activities from the community. They saw the self-help approach as a phase-out strategy. A project approach is evident in this conceptualization of self-help groups: Self-help is utilized as a method of facilitating community participation or as a way of enhancing sustainability of projects conceived and implemented by NGOs.

Sustainability of NGO-sponsored Self-help

There is limited evidence regarding the sustainability of externally sponsored self-help groups (Nayar, Kyobutungi, and Razum, 2004). SEWA has been able to sustain its activities largely because of the intensive inputs and support provided for the maintenance of the groups and due to the evolution of the self-help groups to a more institutionalized form similar to co-operatives. In Bangladesh, one local NGO withdrew from a primary health care project by using the Village Health Development Committees formed in the beginning of the project as a self-help mechanism (Self-help Promotion Secretariat, 2001:26). Although the consequences of the phasing out are not yet clear, it is stated that a phasing out is not impossible if the people are told about it in the beginning of a project. Another NGO promoted a self-reliance strategy because it had previously experienced a sudden withdrawal of donor support. The strategy adopted was the formation of health and management committees with the participation of people. The NGO reports that the task was difficult, as people believed that government and non-government organizations should provide health care free of cost (Self-help Promotion Secretariat, 2001:43-45). In a third case, where health was a major component, a self-sustaining, payment-based card system for free services or a reduction of fees was introduced at the village health posts (Self-help Promotion Secretariat, 2001:59-63). One of the significant limitations identified was the inability to sustain community interest when there were other priorities such as harvesting, or when disasters occurred, for example floods. When self-help is implemented in a project mode, the motivation of the project staff also becomes important. The project staff may have apprehensions about losing their job if the self-help project becomes too successful. In yet another case, self-help was visualized as a community support system for specific problems like obstetric care (Self-help Promotion Secretariat, 2001:74-76). The project tried to link the support system with the local government. Although it found that this approach would potentially increase the access to health care and health information, its sustainability could not be established.

Self-help Under Government Sponsorship

The government of India has adopted the self-help approach and micro-finance programs as tools for women's empowerment, employment generation, and for achieving production-oriented goals. This is part of the overall strategy within the new economic policies to redefine the role of the government (Government of India, 2002d; government of India, 2002e). As discussed in chapter 4, a major initiative, sponsored by the Government and known as "Kudumbashree" (Welfare of the Family), is underway in the state of Kerala. This new scheme, based on the national strategy, is a highly formal and institutionalized approach to self-help. Kudumbashree promotes income generation activities for poor women by organizing Neighborhood Groups (NHG), which will help them to earn higher incomes, thereby enabling them to achieve economic self-sufficiency. Several other state governments in India have also initiated employment programs for women (and even public-limited companies like women's development corporations) based on the concept of self-help. It is hoped that by building community structures of women drawn from poverty-stricken families and by helping them to overcome poverty, social and economic empowerment can be achieved. The empowerment of women gets the central place in the conceptualization of Kudumbashree, although it is operationalized largely through a market-oriented strategy such as micro-enterprises, thrift and credit societies, informal banks, etc.

The health component of Kudumbashree is limited to creating awareness and facilitating access of members to health services (Government of Kerala, *State Poverty Eradication Mission*. http://www.kudumbashree.org; Government of Kerala, undated). Weekly meetings of group members are organized to discuss issues related to hygiene, mother and child care, nutrition, immunization, etc. A community health volunteer who is selected from among the members performs convergence of various programs under the Health and Social Welfare Departments and helps the members, especially women, children and the aged, to access services. A study undertaken in Kerala reveals that the group members are largely involved in only health education activities (Kyobutungi and Nayar, 2005). The members hardly get opportunities to exercise their rights and the activities are limited to income generation and micro-credit. Another study from Kerala shows that micro-credit programs do not offer the background to challenge the inequitable gender relations (Babu, 2011).

Case studies from some other states in India also show that the SHGs have been used to mainly advance micro-finance and income generation for achieving empowerment. Case studies conducted in Bihar, Uttar Pradesh, and Orissa show that micro-credit and micro-finance are not panacea for overall empowerment of women in a society which is dominantly patriarchal (Pandey, 2008; Garg, 2005; Rath, 2009). All the case studies reveal that the prevailing patriarchal social structure precludes women from achieving complete autonomy. Another study conducted in Tamil Nadu shows that although women are more visible due to the SHG and women's entry into politics, they are not to be confused with power and autonomy in decision-making (Lindberg et al., 2011). The study points out that the SHG is a political program which requires vigorous funding as well as NGO support for them to function effectively. As this is subject to political conjectures, they may fade away after the initial enthusiasm.

A Typology of Self-help in South Asia

In Bangladesh and India, three broad scenarios regarding the structure of self-help groups which are involved in some form of health activities are discernible (Nayar, Kyobutungi, Razum, 2004). The characteristics are given in table 5.3. In the two countries, characterized by a hierarchical social structure and a substantial proportion of poor, there is some degree of similarity in the origin of self-help groups: they have not evolved endogenously or as a spontaneous reaction to a common cause, but have been initiated externally. The health-oriented groups in India mainly target women for their programs, resembling the purely market-oriented self-help groups. The NGOs in Bangladesh, on the other hand, are not targeted on women alone. The groups in the two countries follow different approaches and have different emphasis on health issues, from awareness campaigns and health education to primary health care activities as in Bangladesh and the SEWA initiative. However, none of the groups are involved in provision of curative health care, and may not be able to do so considering their composition and focus (except supply of drugs, as in SEWA). The SEWA initiative is characterized by its well-developed organizational structure and intensive inputs, and probably these have helped it to sustain its activities.

Evidence regarding the viability and cost-effectiveness of the self-help approach in health care is limited, partially because of its recent origin. Even SEWA, which has been able to sustain its activities over a longer period, is not a convincing example of alternate community financing in health or provision of good quality clinical care. Moreover, the evidence from Bangladesh shows that self-help has only moderate success as a rollback or phase-out strategy. To some extent, however, self-help groups may be able to increase access to, and facilitate the utilization of, existing health services.

People in Europe and the US form self-help groups to fulfill a need that is not met by existing social and health services. Their aims are multiple and often divergent: to empower themselves; to participate in decision-making; to show concern and compassion for others in an increasingly individualistic society; and to feel being treated as a dignified person, often in response to a health care system that they perceive as high-tech but de-personalized. Given the number and nature of these objectives (which, moreover, may be related to health outcomes only indirectly), the cost-effectiveness of self-help groups has been difficult to evaluate. In consequence, their role in health care provision cannot be considered evidence based. For proponents of self-help groups this is not a problem—they have always insisted that this approach can complement, but never replace, existing health services.

Throughout the history of self-help, there has been a tendency to "usurp" this concept and put it to use in the interest of a conservative political agenda.

Table 5.3. Typology of self-help groups with a health orientation in Bangladesh and India

	Type I: *Limited external assistance*	*Type II:* *Mainly sponsored by NGOs*	*Type III:* *Sponsored by the state*
Approach	Empowerment approach	Empowerment approach. Project approach in some cases	Largely market-oriented at the level of implementation
Orientation	Largely credit and savings	Multi-faceted and development-oriented	Largely production-oriented
Target group	Mainly targeting women	Targeting women and minorities	Targeting women
Health component	Health activities restricted to campaigns	Health activities including focused health programs by some NGO-sponsored groups	Primary health care activities on a limited scale through the community health volunteer
Sustainability	Sustainability not yet demonstrated	Limited evidence of sustainability	Sustainability not yet demonstrated

Source: Nayar et al., 2004

The social Darwinists of the 19th century envisioned a society based on the principle of "survival of the fittest." They demanded "no money for the unfit" and promoted self-help to ease the effect on the poor. In West Germany of the mid-1980s, self-help groups were instrumentalized under a revisionist interpretation of the principle of subsidiarity, again with the outspoken aim to reduce government expenditure, and in spite of missing evidence on cost-effectiveness. Attempts like these ignore that self-help does not come for free (neither for users, nor for the social and health sector), and that it is appropriate only for a small proportion of potential users. The aged, the working, the lower classes, the minority groups are not reached, in other words, the very people that are left most in need when funding of government social and health services is reduced.

In the international health arena today, neo-liberals are trying to appropriate the concept of self-help over again. Self-help groups are being prescribed to alleviate the effects of a utilitarian approach to priority setting in the health sector of developing countries that resulted in "rationing by exclusion" (Stefanini, 1999). Again, it is being overlooked that self-help is not free of cost. Potential users may not be able to afford access to information, transport to reach meetings, the required infrastructure, and clearinghouses to facilitate the formation of new groups, etc. A successful self-help approach requires that lay people not only have access to, but also learn to digest, health-related information that informs their activities. In summary, self-help requires political acceptance and financial support—all at the "risk" of empowering the population! Not only politicians, but also health care professionals have to be compliant. Doctors and nurses need to be prepared to co-operate with clients on an equal basis. This means they need to be involved early on, and be fully convinced of the advantages of self-help approaches, rather than be forced to participate.

In India (Gupta, 2000) and Bangladesh, like in many other developing countries, vertical, hierarchical social structures prevail, creating an environment which is not very encouraging for self-help groups. Given the social structure and the class system prevailing in the Indian society, it may be unrealistic to expect poor women to overcome existing social barriers such as patriarchy just because they have been financially empowered and are trained in leadership activities (Kyobutungi and Nayar, 2005).

In the foregoing analysis, we found that a prescriptive, instrumental approach to self-help is dominant, both in the NGO and the government sector. Judging from experience in Europe, the utility of an approach in which professionals attempt to steer self-help groups from outside is very limited and unlikely to be sustainable, unless continuously supported by considerable financial and organizational inputs. Self-help groups should be voluntary, have a convincing component of service quality assurance, involve doctors early on, and agree upon outcome measures (such as improved health; reduced cost; empowerment) to assess cost-effectiveness.

In order to function, self-help groups require a basic enabling environment such as a stable social structure and a functioning basic health care system offering a minimum standard of quality. The presence of these two factors is a prerequisite for self-help activities; they cannot be expected to develop as a consequence of self-help. Self-help groups can help to achieve some degree of synergy between health care providers and users when the prerequisites mentioned above are met. As long as this is not the case, however, the transfer of a concept that originated in Western, individualistic societies to a very different societal context will bring only disappointing results. Given the evidences available now, under no circumstances self-help groups can fulfill the significant demand for clinical care of good quality in South Asia. Nor can they offer financial protection, i.e., relieve the economic consequences of serious health events occurring at individual or family level. However, they can be involved in facilitating service provision and in strengthening the interphase between community and the health services.

PEOPLE'S MOVEMENTS IN HEALTH

Popular movements and people's action in health have been largely initiated by smaller groups and localized. There are three main categories as identified by Shukla and Phadke (1999). These are: Campaigns for awareness and policy change; initiatives for alternatives and focus on health issues and; groups which focus on research and advocacy. According to them, there are number of organizations involved in health-oriented activities:

- Various people's science groups and consumer groups like KSSP, Delhi Science Forum, Lok Vigyan Sanghatna, ACASH, etc. have been mainly involved in publishing and disseminating materials which have exposed exploitative/irrational activities of the drug industry, unscientific government drug policy, against health-related superstitions, etc.
- The All India Drug Action Network is involved in campaigns for changes in government drug policy with some success.
- Campaigns on women's health issues such as ban on prenatal sex determination have been taken up by women's groups in Maharashtra.
- Professional organizations and trade unions of health functionaries (resident doctors/medical students) have also voiced demands for improvement in health services and supplies in public hospitals and have even expressed concerns regarding unscientific drug policy, etc.

- Some periodicals give a rational, pro-people outlook to a professional audience, notable among which are journals on rational drug therapy like BODHI, BSRT, and drug disease, and doctors. Issues in medical ethics have a similar audience and approach have also received attention.
- The Medico Friend Circle (MFC) is one platform of health activists of various inclinations and backgrounds having functioned continuously over the last 25 years and providing a forum for debate and sharing of ideas relevant to the health movement, namely (Shukla and Phadke, 1999).

CONCLUDING OBSERVATIONS

It can be unequivocally stated that the third options discussed in this chapter, except some exceptions like the people's movements have been appropriated by the neo-liberal agenda as it was assumed that they help in disinvestment and withdrawal of the state from social sectors. It was also assumed that they are more transparent, more efficient, less corrupt, and less bureaucratized than the state. The experience, however, is on the contrary. However, there are a number of lessons one can draw from the experiences of using civil society and especially the third sector organizations or the non-state sector (NSS) for the delivery of services originally intended as state actions. Given the burgeoning role of these actors, there are additional questions as raised by a review undertaken by the Alliance for Health Policy and Systems Research and the WHO (Walker et al., 2009). These are relevant questions to be addressed in the current environment where social sector is being increasingly delegated to such organizations.

1. How can the government create a better environment to foster non-state providers in the achievement of health systems outcomes?
2. What is the quality and / or coverage of health care services provided by the non-state sector for the poor?
3. What types of regulation can improve health systems outcomes, and under what conditions?
4. How best to capture data and trends about private sector providers on a routine basis? (Walker et al., 2009:2)

However, even when it is assumed that the third sector organizations (TSOs) can be an alternative to state for delivering services such as health, there appears to be no reduction in the role of the government. This is due to the nature of the health sector where technology is a major component of the service and the relevance of curative, preventive, and promotive services among the public health activities. Such a comprehensive health services could be delivered in an integrated way only with considerable state-support and investment. Largely due to political compulsions, the neo-liberal reforms could only adopt a partial package of the reduced role of the state and privatization. The imported notion of governance could not be duplicated in the southern countries which had much more complex, hierarchical as well as nuanced socio-political structures and distinct cultural patterns. Secondly, the instrumentalization of the third sector or the non-state Sector, no doubt a reality, only added to the disorder created by the so-called inefficiency of the state. The TSOs and NSS could not surmount the problems due to the same reason stated above.

NOTE

1. This will be further elaborated under the section on cooperatives in health care.

6

Disorder Defined

The Homogenization Process

The disorder in common sense parlor and lexicographically is an antonym of order. The health services, being a component of the society experience disorder which is also embodied in a given socio-political context. Since health services deal with amelioration of disease which itself is a product of bodily disorder and which produces disorder in the individual, family and the society, a socio-cultural and technical entity such as health services is seen as replicating this disorder to some extent. Nevertheless, the disorder-discernible and projected as the maladies of health care in India is to a large extent created by exogenous factors which are sometimes external to the health services as well. One example is the structural adjustment programs and fiscal reforms intended to stabilize the economy impinging on the health services. Therefore, this disorder is not to be analyzed on a scale of lexicographical opposites although it could be critically examined in terms of polarities of conservative and critical public health.

One of the projects of globalization and neo-liberal reforms which is also continuous with past traditions is the *homogenization of order* through organizational strategies, managerial interventions, and technical inputs discussed in the previous chapters which do not respect contextual specificities. This homogenization is sought to be tried through certain procedures, strategies and techniques on the assumptions that the body and the technologies to handle the body are universal and the specific contexts could be ignored. The specificities may be socially and culturally conditioned artifacts including tolerance of ambiguities and disorder. In such a context, the ordering projects may not sustain and may move back to disorder or it may be a slow process. In short, the inefficiencies of public sector health services which is considered as one of the causes of disorder and which are often projected as the rationale for ushering in privatization has to be seen against these specificities. The disorder therefore could be analyzed at different levels. We broadly place this disorder at three levels although further theoretical work can decipher the nuances.

- Disorder emanating from a bureaucratic medicine
- Disorder in medical systems and programs
- Organizational disorder

DISORDER UNDER A BUREAUCRATIC ORDER

The analysis undertaken in the previous chapters revealed an assumption that bureaucratic exercises can bring in both order and stability in health services and enable efficient provisioning of care. The Bhore committee especially has been responsible for such a framework wherein it was thought that a top-down and extremely hierarchical organizational structure using a blueprint approach will help in the universal provisioning of health care to the people. Fundamentally, the question that needs to be raised is the viability and efficacy of providing medical care under such a structure. As subsequent committees, especially the Mudaliar committee noted, the health services that was set-up did not match even a fraction of what the Bhore committee had already visualized and it did not help in taking health care to the doorstep of the people. Evidently, the modern approach as suggested by the Bhore committee was too slow to take root in the country. The state which took up many functions in a centralized way with "ambitious standards of public order and control" could not maintain or sustain them (Hobsbawm, 1994). Obviously, a hierarchical structure with generalists in command of a technical-biomedical service could create problems of dissonance as major decisions regarding the body of a person has to be medically determined in an organization controlled by generalists who have no know-how except for assumptions of rationality and administrative prudence.

The perils of bureaucratic medicine had multiplied because of constant policy shifts due to what can be called as demographic dependency than epidemiological necessity based on priorities. It is now well-known that the family planning program took a heavy toll of whatever organizational credibility the health services had in India. Curtailing population than curtailing ill-health was the preferred organizational imperative of health services. The many committees set-up by the government of India and their influence on health services as reviewed in chapter 2 also played an important role in bureaucratizing the health services as some of them were on a recommendation spree for specific staff patterns with respect to specific vertical programs. This in no small way also created disorder.

There were also silver linings in this bureaucratic disorder. The ICSSR-ICMR committee report is the only exception which at least recommended a more people-oriented system. The report although necessitated by an exogenous event such as the Alma Ata conference gave an indication of the possibility of creating a space where the state, in partnership with the civil society, can take people-centered endogenous actions for achieving health for all and universal health care. The ICSSR-ICMR committee stood apart from the linear-vertical character of many committee recommendations and the recommendations were unlike the instrumental nature of most other committees. Although not completely bureaucratically visualized and operationalized, it was set-up as a follow-up of the Alma Ata conference on primary health care and therefore it was to a large extent influenced by the comprehensive visions and ideals of primary health care. Unfortunately, despite such an integrated vision that existed since the eighties and great clarity regarding universal health care (UHC) and a broader and appropriate conceptualization, universal health currently operationalized in biomedical terms and oriented in service delivery. The universal health care is focusing on provision of care and services and the critical areas for achieving it such as financing, norms, human resources, community participation, access to medicines, vaccines and technology, managerial reforms, etc. are also service-oriented and largely proximal (Nayar, 2013). The continuation of disorder is a possibility writ larger on the face of Indian health services.

DISORDER, MEDICAL SYSTEMS, AND PROGRAMS

The modernization project of the Bhore committee also invented new traditions (Hobswam, 1983) to fit in biomedicine as the dominant medical system in India. Allopathic medicine was considered as a natural choice excluding or ignoring other systems and customs. The strategy and programs were blueprinted which gave little scope for innovation. This also created considerable disorder into the system through which people could ameliorate their health problems by ignoring the plurality of systems available in the country. Health services in India could be considered as a purposive intervention to the existing sub-culture which can be called as a health culture (Banerji,1986). In this perspective "a health problem has to be seen in terms of the dynamics of the biological interactions between the causative agent(s) and a human group against a background of human ecology, which includes cultural, social, economic and political conditions, which influence the natural history of the health problems in that group or community" (Banerji, 1986:147). The choice of medical system(s) therefore has to be in tune with such a socio-cultural complexity. The failure of biomedicine to address the health problems could be partially explained by the misplaced choice of technology.

In recent times, efforts to bring the traditional and alternate systems of medicine under an umbrella of AYUSH (Ayurveda, Yoga, Unani, Sidha, and Homeopathy) into a health service system dominated by biomedicine have been made by the state. The Indian Systems of Medicine now have a larger umbrella to tackle. Obviously, globalization, market preferences, and shifts in world-views toward such systems have played major roles in this decision although in practice these practitioners are reduced into quasi-bureaucrats involved in record-keeping and health campaigns than professionals. Such systems are also hijacked by the market to influence the increasing ranks of middle class who are the consumers of life style products or the beauty products. This could be another style of inventing new traditions which apparently appear to be rooted in traditions but are far removed from the customs of the society. It is also a revaluation of modernity which considers those customs, considered inferior by the modernists have a market potential as they are not considered an obstacle but a resource for taking the capitalist agenda forward (Pieterse, 2001).

The approach for developing health programs was another vehicle for disorder. The dynamics of epidemiology is the starting point for evolving an appropriate approach which is delivered through an agency using a package of technology (Banerji, 1986) that should blend with the pre-existing health culture which is also dynamic in character. Such a systems perspective is the basis of an integrated, interconnected, and comprehensive mechanism for health programs. Evidently, various decisions that are taken to fine tune health services in the country did not adopt such a perspective. This led to mass campaigns based on certain international policy directives and colossal wastage of money in the name of eradication which otherwise could have been done through an integrated disease control strategy.

ORGANIZATIONAL DISORDER

When disorder is further deconstructed, it is possible to state that the constant tinkering of organizational strategies necessitated by international policy changes is a major causal factor. This is also closely linked to the first level, i.e., the bureaucratic medicine. Examples include the family planning program, small-pox eradication, tuberculosis control, pulse-polio program, etc. Health sector reforms and their forms as discussed in chapter 3 added to the misery followed by the National Rural Health Mission which invented new blended and cocktail strategies and approaches. The orthodoxy dominantly believes in the sanctity and success of reforms as long as the state controls the funding. It is assumed that the ownership of provision becomes less important in such a scenario (Hunter, 2008). It is another matter that there is lack of evidence to support this assumption.

As witnessed in the National Health Services in the UK, a number of drawbacks could be observed in India as well regarding unbridled expansion of market co-existing with the public sector (Hunter, 2008). Among these, fragmentation of care between private and public hospitals is emerging as a problem in many urban areas. With the increasing dependence on private sector for institutional care, this could also extend to rural areas. What Hunter calls as "mission creep" for the disparate attempt by the government to regulate market could also extend to hyped actions to achieve targets set by international donor agencies. This could push up untied expenditure by the government as well as increase wasteful expenditure. The current state is called as dysfunctional health services and is termed as one which is "an exemplar of how not to develop and sustain public health services" (PHM, Medact, HAI, MI, TWN, 2011; 104).

In chapter 3, we stated several instances when targeted programs and goals have created disorder in the health services and even the implicit implementation of Millennium Development Goals could also lead to distortions in the comprehensiveness of health services. When the health services adopt a segmented approach as was done for programs such as pulse polio or RCH or the NRHM, it becomes incapable of handling complexities. And the future complexity will be presented in the form of a disease scenario involving both communicable and non-communicable diseases. The emaciated health services would then become increasingly market driven and the present dispensation in the form of public-private partnership will pave the way for such a natural drive for diagnostics and drugs since the non-communicable diseases entail considerable use of the same.

The organizational strategies of the National Rural Health Mission (NRHM) are an amalgamation of the traditional public administration principles anchored on centralization, authority, expertise, and top-down line and command and the new public management anchored on a value for money approach. One can naturally anticipate discordance and disorder in the actual delivery of such a governance structure as politicians will resist reduced control and the dominance of managers. The increasing role of quasi-state organizations also could lead to disorder. In fact, the World Bank had to stop funding for HIV/AIDS anchored on such a quasi-state model due to widespread misappropriation of funds by the NGOs. But whether the NRHM has led to such a situation is an issue which needs further examination but it is possible to predict the high probability and frequency of such situations given the recent experience in the state of Uttar Pradesh.

NEW DOCUMENTATIONS

Against such a scenario of disorder and disjunctions, new international and national policy inclinations seem to be emerging which apparently are intended as remedying actions. The Commission on Social Determinants of Health (CSDH) of the WHO and the High-Level Committee on Universal Health Care of the Planning Commission in India are examples of such intent (WHO, 2008; PHFI, 2011). Both have considerable degree of state and civil society participation and are being discussed in the public domain. However, such intentions need to negotiate with the disordering institutional culture which has resulted from the past policies and actions. In addition, the epidemiological complexity also adds to the disorder. As mentioned earlier in this chapter, mere definitional clarity of the intent is not enough. Universal health care has now become an umbrella goal for the post–2015 development agenda. *Teleologically*, there is a need to ask whether the end product is universal service availability or universal health of the people as there are also moves toward appropriating universal intents to economics and to the reforms framework by identifying financial protection for all from the cost of health care and financing mechanisms as the underlying elements (McIntyre and Mills, 2012; Evans et al., 2013; Kutzin, 2013). This type of conceptualization of UHC has taken the debate to more conventional and conservative public health of considering everything into access which includes physical accessibility, financial affordability, and acceptability (Evans et al., 2013). The need for alleviation of suffering due to health problems is a universal need which is also influenced by the nature of social relationships in hierarchical societies as well as by social and psychological factors. The role of the agency is important but contingent upon the above formulation as *axiomatically*, it is now accepted that health services is only one among many factors which influence health. *Strategically*, therefore, the focus on downstream factors ignoring the more difficult upstream factors compromise universal health. *Technologically*, we need to be concerned about the rampant misuse of machines which preclude universalization. An alternate vision in such a complex context needs to adopt a multi-faceted and multi-dimensional epidemiology with an organizational strategy to ensure equity and emancipation from misery and ill-health.

DISORDER TO STABILITY

Evidently, the Indian state has been subjected to homogenization of order checkmating some enlightened health policy intent which could be reiterated here as the last word. What is problematic in such a homogenization project is the marginalization of critics, criticisms and dissent. Despite such marginalization, a critical discourse on public health has been strong although such alternate visions are often brushed aside by branding them as idealistic. As against this, the dominant academic discourse is closer to the neo-liberal reform agenda and is atheoretical and techno-managerial. Both the reform agenda and this academic discourse assume that the problems of health and health services are the outcome of inefficiency of the government and therefore the solutions lie in reducing the role of the State and increasing the participation of private sector. Such an approach is also similar to the cornucopian stand which assumes that it is possible to correct the deviations by excessive technological inputs and managerial strategies. However, it is necessary to review and reflect on the causes of such inefficiencies and deviations before corrections can be suggested for achieving universal health care. We argue that either such an exercise has not been done or the available counter evidence has not been assessed or they have been ignored in favor of easier downstream factors such as biomedical, behavioral, or educational interventions. We can argue that any policies on universalization of health care should also address the larger societal crises along with interventions in health services.

The larger societal crises in India emerge from the super imposition of the new international capital on a society with wider social differentials. Utsa Patnaik argues, based on the National Sample Survey data that withdrawal of subsidies in agriculture and inability of small and marginal farmers to maintain their livestock as a result of a rise in livestock product price led to increase in landlessness and to enormous loss of livestock. She says that this is not a short-term problem but has been created by an attack on the basic structure of production and the agricultural economy including sharp reduction in public planned development expenditure in rural areas. This agrarian crisis in what she calls as the "Republic of Hunger" (Patnaik, 2004) has also resulted in massive decline in the food grain availability per head from 177 kg in the 1990s to 153 kg in 2003–2004 which is unusual in normal times and not under conflict or disaster conditions. She says that this is a little lower than the 157 kg level during 1937–1941. She also reports that only sub-Saharan African countries and least developed countries have lower levels than this. Neo-liberal reforms have targeted both production and access and such policies have affected the incomes of the farmers thereby also resulting in less employment for the agricultural labor (Patnaik, 2006; Patnaik, 2008). It is quite evident that larger societal crises in India are created by exogenous forces and mediated by indigenous political class. The direct implication of such a crisis on the health of the poor needs no elaboration. As mentioned in chapter 3, there are considerable disparities between different social groups in India with respect to health conditions and health service availability. These disparities continue to exist despite many reforms undertaken in India since the nineties.

This minor digression enables us to reach the central thesis of this book because the larger societal crises act as one of the forces which influence disorder. The central issue that needs to be resolved is the predicament of a teleological understanding of the disorder with respect to health services. The movement is toward stability and not toward order given the disorder inherent in health services. Can there be stability in health services given the existence of larger societal crises? The answer could be obvious but despite such deductive and inductive certainty, the techno-managerial fixes and recommendations and neo-liberal reforms including a movement toward privatization are rampant; ignoring the positive forces within the state and civil society. They are the order of the day! As stated explicitly and implicitly in our earlier chapters, disordered health services—both private and public care and their mix—pushed and pulled by international and national policy intents may not sustain for long and may serve as an inappropriate institutional arrangement to provide universal health and health care. Importantly, stable health services which can ensure equity and equality and thereby universality may emerge only if such larger societal crises such as hunger and poverty are addressed.

References

Alliance for Health Policy and Systems Research. 2004. *Strengthening health systems: the role and promise of policy and systems research*. Geneva: Global Forum for Health Research and WHO.

Araujo, J. Jr., and A. C. Luiz. 1997. "Attempts to decentralize in recent Brazilian health policy: issues and problems, 1988-1994." *International Journal of Health Services* 27: 109-24.

Asian Development Bank. 2002. *Report and recommendation of the President to the Board of Directors on a proposed cluster of loans to India for the Modernizing Government and Fiscal Reform in Kerala program*. Manila: Asian Development Bank.

Attanayake, N. 2001. "An assessment of the effectiveness of decentralization of health services in Sri Lanka." In, *Public Health and the Poverty of Reforms: The South Asian Predicament*, edited by I Qadeer, K. Sen, and K. R. Nayar, 398-412. New Delhi: Sage.

Attwood DW, Baviskar BS. 1998. "Introduction." In, *Who Shares? Cooperatives and Rural Development*, edited by D. W. Attwood, and B. S. Baviskar, 1-20. New Delhi: Oxford University Press.

Aziz, A. 2000. "Democratic decentralization: experience of Karnataka." *Economic and Political Weekly* 35 (39): 3521-3526.

Bambra, C. 2013. "The primacy of politics: the rise and fall of evidence-based public health policy?" *Journal of Public Health 35* (4): 486-87.

Banerji, D. 1982. *Poverty, class and health culture in India*. New Delhi: Prachi Prakashan.

Banerji, D.1985. *Health and family planning services in India: An epidemiological, socio-cultural and political analysis and a perspective*. New Delhi: Lok Paksh.

Banerji, D. 1986. *Social sciences and health service development in India: Sociology of formation of an alternative paradigm*. New Delhi: Lok Paksh.

Bardhan, P. 2002. "Decentralization of governance and development." *The Journal of Economic Perspectives* 16 (4): 185-205.

Basu, SK.1992. "Health and culture among the underprivileged groups in India." In, *State of India's Health*, edited by A. Mukhopadhyay, 175-186. New Delhi: Voluntary Health Association of India.

Beteille, A. 2005. "Civil society and the good society." In, *On civil society: Issues and perspectives*, edited by N. Jayaram, 273-293. New Delhi: Sage.

Bhatt, ER. 1996. "Women's health security: strengthening women's economy." *P.K.Devi Memorial Endowment Oration*. New Delhi: India International Centre.

Bhatt, R. 2000. "Issues in health: public-private partnerships." *Economic and Political Weekly* 35:4706-16.

Bhattacharya, S. S. Messenger, and C. Overy 2010. *Social Determinants of Health: Assessing Theory, Policy and Practice*. Hyderabad: Orient Blackswan.

Birn, Anne-Emanuelle. 2005. "Gates's grandest challenge: transcending technology as public health ideology." *The Lancet* 366: 514-519.

Bloom, G., and G. Xingyuan. 1997. "Health sector reforms: lessons from China." *Social Science and Medicine* 45: 351-60.

Bogg, L., H. Dong, K. Wang, W. Cai, D. Vonod. 1996. "The cost of coverage: rural health insurance in China." *Health and Political Planning* 11: 238-52.

Bossert, T. 1998." Analyzing the decentralization of health systems in developing countries: Decision space, innovation and performance." *Social Science and Medicine* 47 (10): 1513-27.

Bowen, S., and A. B. Zwi. 2005. Pathways to 'evidence-informed' policy and practice: A framework for action. *PLoS medicine* 2 (7): 600-605.

Carrin, G., A. Ron, Y. Hui, W. Hong, Z. Tuohong, Z. Licheng, Z. Shuo, Y. Yide, C. Jiaying, J. Qicheng, Z. Zhaoyang, Y. Jun, and L. Xuesheng. 1999. "The reform of the rural cooperative medical system in the People's Republic of China: interim experience in 14 pilot counties." *Social Science and Medicine* 48: 961-72.

Cassels, A. 1995. "Health Sector Reform: Key issues in less developed countries. Discussion Paper No.." Geneva: WHO.

Chambers, R., and G. V. Medeazza. 2013. "Sanitation and stunting in India: Undernutrition's blind spot." *Economic and Political Weekly* 48 (25): 15-18.

Chase, E., and R. Carr-Hill. (1994). "The dangers of managerial perversion: quality assurance in primary health care." *Health Policy and Planning* 9 (3): 267-278.

Chuengsatiansup, K. 2008. *Deliberative action: civil society and health systems reform in Thailand*. Nonthaburi: National Health Commission Office.

Coffey, D., A. Deaton, J. Dreze, et. al, 2013 "Stunting among children: facts and implications." *Economic and Political Weekly* 48(34):68-70.

Collins, C., and A. Green.1994. "Decentralization and primary health care: some negative implications in developing countries." *International Journal of Health Services* 24: 459-75.

CSDH. 2008. *Closing the gap in a generation: health equity through action on the Social Determinants of Health. Final Report of the Commission on Social Determinants of Health*. Geneva: World health Organization.

Daar, A. S., P. A. Singer, D. L. Persad, S. K. Pramming, D. R. Matthews, R. Beaglehole, A. Bernstein, L. K. Borysiewicz, S. Colagiuri, N. Ganguly, R. I. Glass, D. T. Finegood, J. Koplan, E. G. Nabel, G. Sarna, N. Sarrafzadegan, R. Smith, D. Yach, and J. Bell. 2007. "Grand challenges in chronic non-communicable diseases: The top 20 policy and research priorities for conditions such as diabetes, stroke and heart disease." *Nature* 450: 494-96.

Das, A., D. Rao, A. Hagopian. 2011. "India's Janani Suraksha Yojana: further review needed." *The Lancet* 377: 295-96.

Das, J., and J. Leino. 2011. " Evaluating the RSBY: lessons from an experimental information campaign." *Economic and Political Weekly* 45 (32): 85-93.

Das, M. K. 2000. "Kerala's decentralized planning: Floundering experiment." *Economic and Political Weekly* 35 (49): 4300-4303

Das, V., R. K. Das, L. Coutinho. 2000. "Disease control and immunisation: a sociological enquiry." *Economic and Political Weekly* 35 (8 and 9): 625-632.

Djurfeldt, G., and S. Lindberg. 1976. *Pills against poverty: a study of the introduction of western medicine in a Tamil village*. New Delhi: Oxford and IBH Publishing Company.

Doherty, J., and L. Gilson. 2006. *Proposed areas of investigation for the KN: an initial scoping of the literature. Health Systems Knowledge Network. Discussion Document No. 1*. Geneva: WHO.

Dreze, J., and A. Sen. 2002. "Democratic practice and social inequality in India." *Journal of Asian and African Studies* 37 (2): 6-37.

Dubos, R. 1965. *Man adapting*. New Haven: Yale University Press.

Dubos, R. 1968. *Man, medicine and environment*. Harmondsworth: Penguin.

Dubowitz, T., D. Levinson, J. N Peterman, G. Verma, S. Jacob, and W. Schultink. 2007. "Intensifying efforts to reduce child malnutrition in India: An evaluation of the Dular program in Jharkhand, India." *Food and Nutrition Bulletin* 28 (3) :266-273.

ECCP project. 2005. *Strengthening micro health insurance units for the poor in India. Position paper submitted to the Parliamentary Committee on Public Undertakings Hearing on health insurance*. New Delhi: Micro Insurance Academy.

Edwards, M. 1999. "Legitimacy and values in NGOs and voluntary organizations: Some skeptical thoughts." In, *International perspectives on voluntary action: Reshaping the third sector*, edited by D. Lewis, 258-267. London: Earthscan.

Estes, C. L , and K. W. Linkins.1997. "Devolution and aging policy: racing to the bottom in long-term care." *International Journal of Health Services* 27: 427-42.

European Union and Government of Chattisgarh. 2011. *Draft Report on evaluation of Community Health Volunteer (Mitanin) Program*. Raipur: Department of Health

Evans, D. B., J. Hsu, and T. Boerma. 2013. "Universal health coverage and universal Access." *Bulletin of the World Health Organization* 91:546–546A

Feng, X., S. Tang, G. Bloom, M. Segall, and Y. Gu. 1995. "Cooperative medical schemes in contemporary China." *Social Science and Medicine* 41: 1111-1118.

Fishbein, M. 2000. "The role of theory in HIV prevention." *AIDS care* 12 (3): 273-278.

Franco, T. D., and K. Kalpana. 1999. *United we sit*. New Delhi: Bharat Gyan Vigyan Samiti.

Friberg, P., S. Wall, Y. Blomstedt, R. Beaglehole, R. Bonita, G. Stordalen, P. Byass. 2012. "Public and global engagement with global health." *The Lancet* 381: 2066.

Friel, S., and P. I. Baker. 2009. "Equity, food security and health equity in the Asia Pacific region." *Asia Pacific Journal of Clinical Nutrition* 18(4):620-632.

Gautam, M., and K. M. Shyamprasad. 2010. The 'basic doctor' for rural India: A failed promise. *Economic and Political Weekly* 45 (38): 25-29.

George, J. 2003. *Decentralised administration and participatory planning in Kerala.* Mumbai: Himalaya Publishing House.

George, M. V. 1976. "A community approach to health care services by popularising cooperative rural dispensaries." In, *Alternative approaches to health care: report of a symposium organised jointly by ICMR and ICSSR.*" New Delhi: Indian Council of Medical Research

George, S. 1994. *Matter of people: co-operative dairying in India and Zimbabwe.* New Delhi: Oxford University Press.

Global HIV prevention working group . 2008. "Behavior change and HIV prevention: (Re) considerations for the 21st century." Accessed 25/07/2013 http://www.globalhivprevention.org.

Gopalan, C. 2013. "The changing nutrition scenario." *Indian Journal of Medical Research*138: 392-397.

Government of Chattisgarh. 2012. Accessed 29 July. http://health.cg.gov.in/ehealth/welcome.htm.

Government of Gujarat. 2012. Accessed 30 Jul. http://www.gujaratindia.com.

Government of India. 1946. *Report of the health survey and development committee (Bhore Committee) Vol. II and IV.* Delhi: Manager of Publications.

Government of India. 1960. *Some Successful Cooperatives – Case Studies. PEO Study No.35.* New Delhi: Program Evaluation Organization, Planning Commission.

Government of India. 1962. *Report of the health survey and planning committee (Mudaliar committee). Vol. I.* Delhi: Manager of publications.

Government of India. 1962. *Report of the health survey and planning committee (Mudaliar committee). Vol. II. Appendices.* Delhi: Manager of publications.

Government of India. 1963. *Report of the special committee on the preparation for entry of the national malaria eradication programme into the maintenance phase (Chadha committee).* New Delhi: Directorate General of Health Services, Ministry of Health.

Government of India. 1966. *Report on I.U.C.D. (Mukerji committee).* New Delhi: Central Family Planning Council.

Government of India. 1966. *Report on basic health services.* New Delhi: Ministry of Health.

Government of India. 1967. *Report of the committee on integration of health services (Jungalwalla committee).* New Delhi: Directorate General of Health Services.

Government of India. 1973. *Report of the committee on multi-purpose workers (Kartar Singh committee).* New Delhi: Ministry of Health and Family Planning.

Government of India. 1976. *Health services and medical education—A programme for immediate action. Report of the group on medical education and support manpower (Shrivastav committee).* New Delhi: Ministry of Health and Family Planning.

Government of India. 1981, Report *of the working group on health for all by 2000 AD*. New Delhi: Ministry of Health and Family Welfare.

Government of India. 1983a. *National health policy*. New Delhi: Ministry of Health and Family Welfare.

Government of India.1983b. *Central Council of Health and Family Welfare: Report of the 9th Joint conference: Agenda notes, Vol. 2*. New Delhi: Ministry of Health and Family Welfare.

Government of India. 1987. *Expert Committee on Health Manpower Planning, Production and Management* (*Bajaj Committee*). New Delhi: Government of India.

Government of India. 1993. *The Constitution Seventy Third Amendment Act, 1992. The Gazette of India Extraordinary 1993. Part II, Section I. No. 69*. New Delhi: Ministry of Law, Justice, and Company Affairs.

Government of India. 1999. *Functioning of Community Health Centres*. New Delhi: Programme Evaluation Organization, Planning Commission.

Government of India. 2001. *Approach Paper to the Tenth Five Year Plan (2002-2007*). New Delhi: Planning Commission.

Government of India. 2001a. *Evaluation Study on Functioning of Primary Health Centres(PHCs) Assisted under Social Safety Net Program (SSNP)*. New Delhi: Planning Commission.

Government of India. 2001b. *Approach Paper to the 10th Five Year Plan (2002-2007)*. New Delhi: Planning Commission.

Government of India. 2002a. *Report of the committee on India Vision 2020*. New Delhi: Planning Commission.

Government of India. 2002b. *National health policy*. New Delhi: Ministry of Health and Family Welfare.

Government of India. 2002c. *10th five year plan, Vol.2, Chapter 2.8, Health*. New Delhi: Planning Commission.

Government of India 2002d. "Ninth Five Year Plan." Accessed 14 Feb. http://planningcommission.nic.in/fiveyr/welcome.html.

Government of India. 2002e. Department of Women and Child Development. "National policy on women empowerment." Accessed 18 Feb. http://wcd.nic.in.

Government of India. 2002f. "Annual report 1999-2000," Accessed 10 July. http://mohfw.nic.in/reports/1999-20Er/Contents.pdf

Government of India. 2002g. "Performance budget. 1999-2000." Accessed10 July. http://mohfw.nic.in/reports/1999-20Epb/CONTENTS.pdf.

Government of India, Planning Commission. 2004. "9th five year plan." Accessed 3 Jan. http://planningcommission.nic.in/plans/planrel/fiveyr/default.html.

Government of India. 2005. *Report of the National Commission on Macroeconomics and Health*. New Delhi: Ministry of Health and Family Welfare.

Government of India. 2006a. *Maternal Mortality in India: 1997-2003 Trends, Causes and Risk Factors* . New Delhi: Registrar General of India.

Government of India. 2006b. *Draft report of the reconstituted task group on public private partnership under NRHM*. New Delhi: Ministry of Health and Family Welfare.

Government of India. 2007. *Guidelines: Central Rural Sanitation Program—Total Sanitation Campaign*. New Delhi: Ministry of Rural Development.

Government of India. 2008. Accessed 4 March http://mohfw.nic.in/NRHM/RCH/Background_new.htm#

Government of India. 2009a. *Special Bulletin on Maternal Mortality in India: 2004-06*. New Delhi: Registrar General of India.

Government of India. 2009b. *National Health Accounts*. New Delhi: Ministry of Health and Family Welfare.

Government of India. 2010. *Annual report to the people on health*. New Delhi: Ministry of Health and Family Welfare.

Government of India. 2010a. *National Rural Drinking Water Program: movement towards ensuring people's drinking water security in rural India*. New Delhi: Ministry of Rural Development.

Government of India. 2011. *Fourth Common Review Mission Report 2010*. New Delhi: NRHM, Ministry of Health and Family Welfare.

Government of India. 2011a. *Special Bulletin on Maternal Mortality in India: 2007-09*. New Delhi: Registrar General of India.

Government of India. 2011b. *Report of the working group on disease burden for 12th five year plan. WG- 3 (2), Non-Communicable Diseases*. New Delhi: Planning Commission.

Government of India. 2011c. *Report of the working group on disease burden for 12th five year plan. WG- 3 (1), Communicable Diseases*. New Delhi: Planning Commission

Government of India. 2011d. *Fourth Common Review Mission Report 2010*. New Delhi: NRHM, Ministry of Health and Family Welfare.

Government of India. 2012a. *Indian Public Health Standards (IPHS): Guidelines for Sub Centres. Revised*. New Delhi: Ministry of Health and Family Welfare.

Government of India. 2012b. *Indian Public Health Standards (IPHS): Guidelines for Primary Health Centres*. New Delhi: Ministry of Health and Family Welfare.

Government of India. 2012c. *Indian Public Health Standards (IPHS): Guidelines for Community Health Centres*. New Delhi: Ministry of Health and Family Welfare

Government of India. 2012d. *Indian Public Health Standards (IPHS): Guidelines for Sub district/sub divisional hospitals (30 to 100 bedded)*. New Delhi: Ministry of Health and Family Welfare.

Government of India. 2012e. *Indian Public Health Standards (IPHS: Guidelines for district hospitals (101 to 500 bedded)*. New Delhi: Ministry of Health and Family Welfare

Government of India, 2013 "SRS bulletins." Accessed 4 March. http://censusindia.gov.in/vital_statistics/SRS_Bulletins/Bulletins.aspx

Government of Kerala. 1997. *People's planning*. Trivandrum: The Planning Board.

Government of Kerala. 1998. *Study report of the committee on cooperative hospitals and dispensaries*. Trivandrum: Registrar of Cooperative Societies.

Government of Kerala. 2002. "State Poverty Eradication Mission." Accessed 14 Feb. http://www.kudumbashree.org

Government of Kerala. undated. State Poverty Eradication Mission. Trivandrum: Kudumbashree Media Division.

Government of Madhya Pradesh. 2012. Accessed 29 Jul. http://www.health.mp.gov.in/healthpolicy.htm

Government of Madhya Pradesh. 2012a. Accessed 29 Jul. http://www.health.mp.gov.in/nrhm.htm

Government of Odisha. undated. Tribal health . Bhubaneswar: NRHM

Government of Uttar Pradesh. 2008. *Behaviour Change Communication (BCC) strategy for NRHM in Uttar Pradesh*. Lucknow: Department of Health and Family Welfare.

Green, A., and A. Matthias. 1997. *Non governmental organizations and health in Developing Countries*. Hampshire and London: Macmillan Press.

Gulati A., A. Ganesh-Kumar, G. Shreedhar, and T. Nandakumar . 2012. "Agriculture and malnutrition in India." *Food and Nutrition Bulletin*, 33 (1): 74-86

Gunatilleke, G. 1984. Ed. *Intersectoral linkages and health development: Case studies in India (Kerala State), Jamaica, Norway, Sri Lanka and Thailand. WHO Offset Publication No.83*, Geneva: World Health Organization.

Gupta, D. 2000. *Mistaken modernity: India between worlds*. New Delhi: HarperCollins Publishers India.

Gupta, A., B. Patnaik, D. Singh, et. al, 2013. "Are child malnutrition figures for India exaggerated?" *Economic and Political Weekly* 48:73-77.

Hanson, K., L. Archard, and B .McPake. 2001. "Creating markets in hospital care: the adoption of developed country health sector reforms by developing countries. Is it appropriate?" *Tropical Medicine and International Health* 6: 747-8.

Hao, Y., H. Lucas, G. Xing-Yuan, and S. Bao-Gang. 1998. *Financing health care in poor rural counties in China: Experience from a township-based co-operative medical scheme. IDS Working Paper 66*. Sussex: Institute of Development Studies.

Helliwell, J., R. Layard, and J. Sachs. 2012. *World Happiness Report*. Columbia: The Earth Institute, Columbia University.

Hobsbawm, E. J. 1983. "Introduction: Inventing Traditions." In, *The invention of Tradition*, edited by EJ Hobsbawm, and T. Ranger, 1-14. Cambridge: Cambridge University Press.

Hobsbawm, E. J. 1994. *The age of extremes: The short twentieth century*. London: Abacus.

Holst, J. 2006. "User fees in health care: myths, truths and evidences." In, *Financing health care—a dialogue between South Eastern Europe and Germany*, edited by U Laaser, and R Radermacher, 69-114. Dusseldorf: Jacobs-Verlag.

Hsiao, W. C. 2004. "Experience of community health financing in the Asian region." In, *Health financing for poor people: resource mobilization and risk sharing*, edited *by* A. S. Preker, and G. Carrin, 119-156. Washington DC: The World Bank.

Hsiao, W. C., and P. S. Heller. 2007. "What should macro-economists know about health care policy?" *International Monetary Fund Working paper series WP/07/13*.

Hunter, D. J. 2008. *The health debate*. Bristol: The Policy Press.

Huss R., A. Green, H. Sudarshan, S. Karpagam, K. Ramani, G. Tomson, and N. Gerein. 2011. "Good governance and corruption in the health sector: Lessons from the Karnataka experience." *Health Policy and Planning* 26: 471-84.

Hussi, P., J. Murphy, O. Lindberg, and L., Brenieman, 1993. *The development of co-operatives and other rural organizations: The role of the World Bank. World Bank Technical Paper series 199*. Washington: The World Bank.

Hutchinson, L., and A. K. LaFond. 2004. *Monitoring and evaluation of decentralization reforms in developing country health sectors*. Bethesda, MD: The Partners for Health Reform plus Project.

Hyden, G. 1988. "Approaches to cooperative development: blueprint versus greenhouse." In, *Who Shares? Cooperatives and Rural Development*, edited by D. W. Attwood, and B. S. Baviskar, 149-71. New Delhi: Oxford University Press.

ICSSR-ICMR. 1980. *Health for all: An alternative strategy*. Pune: Indian Institute of Education.

International Co-operative Information Centre. Undated. *Co-operatives in the health sector. The International Co-operative Movement and the World Summit for Social Development, Background Information 6*. Geneva: International Co-operative Information Centre.

International Institute for Population Sciences, 1995, *National Family Health Survey (MCH and Family Planning), 1992–93, India*. Bombay: IIPS.

International Institute for Population Sciences and ORC Macro, 2000, *National Family Health Survey (NFHS-2), 1998–99, Government of India*. Mumbai: IIPS.

International Institute for Population Sciences, 2007, *National Family Health Survey (NFHS-3), 2004–05, Government of India*. Mumbai: IIPS.

Irwin, L. G., A. Siddiqi, and C. Hertzman. 2007. *Early child development: A powerful equalizer. Final report for the WHO's Commission on Social Determinants of Health*. Geneva: World Health Organization, Commission on Social Determinants of Health.

Jaffri, A. 2001. "Promises and problems of Panchayati Raj: experiences from Madhya Pradesh." In, *Public Health and the Poverty of Reforms: The South Asian Predicament*, edited by I. Qadeer, K. Sen, and K. R. Nayar, 379-397. New Delhi: Sage.

James, K. S. 2007. "Decentralization and its impact on health in India: A review of evidence." In, *Local governance in India: Ideas, challenges and strategies*, edited by P. M. Mathew, 155-177. New Delhi: Concept Publishing Company.

Jayaseelan, J. 1993. "Responding to local needs. Self-help groups." *AIDS Action* 20: 4.

Jeffrey, P., and R. Jeffrey. (2010). "Only when the boat has started sinking: A maternal death in rural North India." *Social Science and Medicine* 71 (10):1711-1718.

Jhabvala, R., and N. Bali. Undated. *My life my work: a sociological study of SEWA's urban members. Working Paper No.2*. Ahmedabad: SEWA Academy,.

Jobert, B. 1985. "Populism and health policy: the case of community health volunteers in India." *Social Science and Medicine* 20: 1-28.

Karmakar, K. G. 1999. *Rural credit and self-help groups: micro-finance needs and Concepts in India*. New Delhi: Sage.

Katz, A. H. 1981. "Self-help and mutual aid: An emerging social movement?" *Annual Review of Sociology* 7: 29-55.

Kaviraj, S. 2001. "In search of civil society." In, *Civil society: history and possibilities*, edited by S. Kaviraj, and S. Khilnani, 287-323. New Delhi: Cambridge University Press.

Kawanga, M. 2005. "Decentralization of health systems." In, *The right reforms? Health sector reforms and sexual and reproductive health,* edited by T. K. S Ravindran, and H. de Pinho, 172-214. South Africa: Women's Health Project, School of Public Health, University of the Witwatersrand.

Khilnani, S. 2001. "The development of civil society." In, *Civil society: history and possibilities*, edited by S. Kaviraj, and S. Khilnanai, 11-32. New Delhi: Cambridge University Press.

Kilby, P. 2011. *NGOs in India: the challenges of women's empowerment and accountability*. London and NY: Routledge.

Kothari, R. 1996. "Issues in decentralized governance." In, *Decentralized governance in Asian countries*, edited by A. Aziz, and D. Arnold, 34-41. New Delhi: Sage.

Krieger, N. 2001. "Theories of social epidemiology in the 21st century: an ecosocial perspective." *International Journal of Epidemiology* 30: 668-677.

Krieger, N. 2005. "Introduction." In, *Health disparities and the body politic*, edited by M. Drexler, 5-9. Boston, Massachusetts: Harvard School of Public Health. pp. 5-9.

Krieger, N. 2005. "Embodiment: a conceptual glossary for epidemiology." *Journal of Epidemiology and Community Health* 59: 350-355.

Krieger, N. 2008. "Proximal, Distal, and the politics of causation: what's level got to do with it?." *American Journal of Public Health* 98 (2): 221-230.

Krishnamurty, H. R. 2013. "Behavioural change towards healthy life styles is the key to check diabetes Under NPCDCS." Accessed 9 November. http://pib.nic.in/newsite/efeatures.aspx?relid=87832.

KSSP. 2006. *Kerala Padanam (in Malayalam)*. Trivandrum: Kerala Sashtra Sahitya Parishad.

Kutzin, J. 2013. "Health financing for universal coverage and health system performance: concepts and implications for policy." *Bulletin of the World Health Organization* 91: 602-611.

Kyobutungi, C., and K. R. Nayar. 2005. "Community participation in health: a qualitative study of women's self-help groups in Kerala state, India." *Journal of Health and Development* 1 (4): 91-102.

Lagarde, M., A. Haines, and N. Palmer. 2009. *The impact of conditional cash transfers on health outcomes and use of health services in low and middle income countries: Review*. Cochrane Collaboration, John Wiley and Sons. Accessed 27-10-2012. http://www.thecochranelibrary.com

Lewis, D. 1999. "Introduction: The parallel universes of third sector research and the changing context of voluntary action." In, *International perspectives on voluntary action: Reshaping the third sector*, edited by D Lewis, 1-17. London: Earthscan.

Lim, S. S., D Lalit, J. A. Hoisington, S. L. James, M. C. Hogan, and E. Gakidou. 2010. "India's Janani Suraksha Yojana, a conditional transfer programme to increase births in health facilities: an impact evaluation." *The Lancet* 375: 2009-2023.

Lindberg, S., V. B. Athreya, R. Vidyasagar, G. Djurfeldt, A. Rajagopal. 2011. "A silent revolution? Women's empowerment in rural Tamil Nadu." *Economic and Political Weekly* 46 (13): 111-120.

Liu, X.Z., and J. L. Wang. 1991. "An introduction to China's health care system." *Journal of Public Health Policy* 12 (1):104-16.

Liu, X., and H. Cao. 1992. "China's cooperative medical system: its historical transformation and the trend of development." *Journal of Public Health Policy* 13: 501-11.

Liu, Y., S. Hu, W. Fu, W. C. Hsiao. 1996. "Is community financing necessary for rural China?" *Health Policy* 38: 155-71.

Mahipal. 2004. "Panchayati raj and rural governance: Experience of a decade." *Economic and Political Weekly* 39 (2): 137-143.

Marmot, M. 1999. "Introduction." In, *Social determinants of health*, edited by M. Marmot, and R. G. Wilkinson, 1-16. Oxford: Oxford University Press.

Mathew, G. 1998. *Panchayati Raj: from legislation to movement*. New Delhi: Concept Publishing company.

Mathur, K. 1998. "Challenges of decentralization: The politics of Panchayati Raj." In, *People's power and Panchayati Raj: theory and practice*, edited by SJSL Raj, and E. Mathias, 1-18. New Delhi; Indian Social institute.

Mayoux, L. 2001. "From vicious to virtuous circles? Gender and micro-enterprise development." Occasional Paper Number 3, U.N. Fourth World Conference on Women. Accessed 14-02-2001 http://www.unrisd.org/engindex/publ/list/opb/opb3/opb3- 03.html

McIntyre, D., and A. Mills. 2012. "Research to support universal coverage in Africa: the SHIELD project." *Health Policy and Planning* 27: i1-i3.

McKeown, T. 1976. *The modern rise of population*. London: Edwin Arnold.

Michaud C., and C. J. L Murray. 1994. "External assistance to the health sector in developing countries: a detailed analysis," 1972-90." *Bulletin of the World Health Organization* 72 (4):639-51.

Mishra US (2011). "Equity implication of health sector decentralization: The case of Kerala state" India. Accessed 21December. www.hsph.harvard.edu/research/takemi/files/RP222.pdf

Mladovsky, P., and E. Mossialos. 2006. *A conceptual framework for community-based health insurance in low-income countries: social capital and economic development. Working Paper No. 2/2006*. London: London School of Economics and Political Science.

Montagu, D. D., A Anglemyer, M. Tiwari, K. Drasser, G. W. Rutherford, T. Horvath, G. E. Kennedy, L. Bero, N. Shah, and H. S. Kinlaw. 2011. *Private versus public strategies for health service provision for improving health outcomes in resource-limited settings.* San Francisco: Global Health Sciences, University of California, San Francisco.

Moore, M. 1996. *Public sector reform: Downsizing, restructuring, improving performance. Discussion Paper No. 7.* Geneva: World Health Organization, Forum on Health Sector Reform.

Mukherjee, N., and D. Bandopaddhyay. 1995. "New horizons for West Bengal panchayats: A report for the Government of West Bengal." *Indian Journal of Agricultural Economics* 50 (4): 688-98.

Mukhopadhyay, A. 2007. "South Asia's health promotion kaleidoscope." *Promotion & Education*14 (4): 238-243.

Mushtaque, A., R. Chowdhury, and A. Bhuiya. 2001. "Do poverty alleviation programs reduce inequities in health? The Bangladesh experience." In, *Poverty, in-*

equality and health: an international perspective, edited *by* DA Leon, and G Walt, 313-331. Oxford: Oxford University Press.

Mykhalovskiy, E., and L. Weir. 2004. "The problems of evidence-based medicine: directions for social science." *Social Science and Medicine* 59: 1059-1069.

Naidoo, K., and R. Tandon. 1999. "The promise of civil society." In, *Civil society at the millennium*, edited by CIVICUS, 1-16. Connecticut: Kumarian Press.

Nambiar, ACK. 1996. "New frontiers in co-operation: Co-operative hospitals in Kerala." In, *Rediscovering co-operation – Co-operatives in the emerging context Vol.3*, edited by R. Rajagopalan, 118-36. Anand, Gujarat: Institute of Rural Management.

Narayana, D. 2010. "Review of Rashtriya Swasthya Bima Yojana." *Economic and Political Weekly* 45 (29): 13-18.

National Planning Committee. 1948. *Report of the subcommittee on national health (Sokhey Committee).* Bombay: Vora & Company publishers Limited.

National Planning Committee. 1948b. *Report of the subcommittee on national housing (Prabhavalkar Committee).* Bombay: Vora & Company publishers Limited.

Navarro, V. 1976. *Medicine under capitalism*. New York: Prodist

Navarro, V., and L. Shi. 2001. "The political context of social inequalities and health." *Social Science and Medicine* 52 : 481-91.

Nayar, K. R. 1987. "Housing in rural areas: a social science perspective." *State and Society* 7 (3): 30-39.

Nayar, K. R. 1993. "Social sciences in health: towards a paradigm." *IASSI Quarterly*12 (1&2): 153-159

Nayar, K. R. 1996. "Housing water supply and sanitation: an assessment of problems and prospects." *IASSI Quarterly* 14 (1 & 2): 103-109.

Nayar, K. R. 1998. "Old priorities and new agenda of public health in India: is there a mismatch?" *Croatian Medical Journal* 39 (3): 308-315.

Nayar, K. R. 2000. "Decline of co-operative medical services in Kerala." *Economic and Political Weekly* 35 (7): 519-21.

Nayar, K. R. 2000. "Public medicare: unhealthy trends." *Economic and Political Weekly* 35 (31): 2699-2700.

Nayar, K. R. 2001. Politics of decentralization: Lessons from Kerala. In, *Public health and the poverty of reforms: the South Asian predicament*, edited by I. Qadeer, K. Sen, and K. R. Nayar, 363-378. New Delhi: Sage.

Nayar, K. R., C. Kyobutungi, and O. Razum. 2004. "Self-help: what future role in health care for low and middle-income countries?" *International Journal for Equity in Health* 3 (1):1.

Nayar, K. R., and O. Razum. 2006. "Millennium Development Goals and health: another selective development?" *International Studies* 43 (3): 317-22.

Nayar, K. R., and S. Nair. 2006. "Kerala's roadmap to privatization in health care." *Journal of Health and Development* 2 (1 and 2): 43-50.

Nayar, K. R., and Ritu Priya. 2007. "Critical public health: operationalising a vision." *MFC Bulletin* 323-324: 40-44.

Nayar, K. R. 2011. "Gaps in goals: The history of goal-setting in health care in India." *Oman Medical Journal* 26 (1): 1-3.

Nayar, K. R. 2011. "India's country experience in addressing social exclusion in maternal and child health," *Country case study No.8.* Geneva: WHO. CSDH.

Nayar, K. R. 2012. "Three decades of ICSSR-ICMR Committee Report & the reassertion of social determinants of health." *Indian Journal of Medical Research* 136: 540-543.

Nayar, K. R. 2013. *Intersectoral approach and health in All (HiA) policies in South East Asia Region.* New Delhi: WHO SEARO Regional paper.

Nayar, K. R. 2013. "Universalizing health care in India: the techno-managerial fix." *Indian Journal of Public Health* 57 (4): 76-81.

Nayar, K. R. 2014. "Inclusion and empowerment in maternal health services in India: An analysis of new initiatives." *Santhigiri Synthesis: Research Paper Series No.1.* Thiruvananthapuram: Santhigiri Social Research Institute.

Nayar, P. K. B. 2005. "Civil society, state and democracy: lessons for India." In, *On civil society: Issues and perspectives*, edited by N Jayaram, 124-136. New Delhi: Sage.

Osborne, K. 1997. "Support to HIV-positive people, NAPWA South Africa." *AIDS Bull.* 6: 38-39.

Palacios, R. 2010. "A new approach to providing health insurance to the poor in India: The early experience of Rashtriya Swasthya Bima Yojna. RSBY Working paper 1." Accessed 9-3-2012 http://www.rsby.gov.in/Documents.aspx?ID=14

Panagariya, A. 2013. "Does India really suffer from worse child malnutrition than Sub-Saharan Africa?" *Economic and Political Weekly*, 48)18):98-111.

Panikkar, P. G. K., and C. R. Soman. 1984. *Health status of Kerala: Paradox of economic backwardness and health development.* Trivandrum: Centre for Development Studies.

Patnaik, U. 2004. "The republic of hunger." *Public lecture on the occasion of 50th birth anniversary of Safdar Hasmi, April 10 2004.* New Delhi: SAHMAT.

Patnaik, U. 2006. "Poverty and neo-liberalism in India." *Rao Bahadur Kale Memorial Lecture, February 3 2006*, Pune: Gokhale Institute of Politics and Economics.

Patnaik, U. 2008. "Theorizing poverty and food security in the era of economic reforms." In, *Globalization and the Washington consensus: its influence on democracy and development in the South*, edited by D. Lechini, 161-200. Buenos Aires: CLACSO.

PHFI. 2011. *High Level Expert Group Report on Universal Health Coverage for India.* New Delhi: Public Health Foundation of India.

PHM, Medact, HAI, MI, TWN. 2011. *Global health watch: an alternative world health report.* New York: Zed Books.

Pieterse, J. N. 2001. *Development theory: deconstructions/reconstructions.* New Delhi: Vistaar Publications.

Perez, E., J. Cardosi, Y. Coombes, J. Devine, A. Grossman, C. Kullmann, C. A. Kumar, N. Mukherjee, M. Prakash, A. Robiarto, D. Setiawan, U. Singh, and D. Wartono. 2012. *What does it take to scale up rural sanitation?* Washington: Water and Sanitation Program.

Prasad, N. P. and P. Raghavendra. 2012. "Healthcare models in the era of medical neo-liberalism: a study of Aarogyasri in Andhra Pradesh." *Economic and Political Weekly* 47 (43): 118-126.

Preker, A. S., G. Carrin, D. Dror, M. Jakab, W. Hsiao, and D. Arhin-Tenkorang. 2002. "Effectiveness of community health financing in meeting the cost of illness." *Bulletin of the World Health Organization* 80:143-150.

Purdom, W. 1973. Ed. *Environmental health.* New York: Academic Press.

Purohit, B. C. 2001. "Private initiatives and policy options: recent health system experience in India." *Health Policy and Planning*16: 87-97.

Qadeer, I., K. Sen, and K. R. Nayar. 2001. eds. *Public health and the poverty of reforms: the South Asian predicament.* New Delhi: Sage.

Qadeer, I. 2001. "Impact of structural adjustment programs on concepts in public health." In, *Public health and the poverty of reforms: the South Asian predicament*, edited by I. Qadeer, K. Sen, and K. R. Nayar, 117-136. New Delhi: Sage.

Qadeer, I., and K. R. Nayar. 2005. "Politics of pedagogy in public health." *Social Scientist* 33 (1-2): 47-75.

Qadeer, I. 2005. "Population control in the era of neo-liberalism." *Journal of Health and Development* 1 (4): 31-48.

Qadeer, I., and R. Dasgupta. 2007. "Planning for primary health care within the National Rural Health Care in India." *Journal of Health and Development* 3 (3and 4); 7-27.

Qadeer, I. 2011. *Public health in India: critical reflections.* New Delhi: Daanish Publishers.

Rajagopal. 1999. "Empowering rural women's groups for strengthening economic linkages: some Indian experiments." *Development in Practice* 9: 327-341.

Ramachandran, P. 2013. Food and nutrition security: challenges in the new millennium. *Indian Journal of Medical Research* 138: 373-382.

Rao, S .1994. ed. *Panachayti Raj and health. Proceedings of the seminar, 9-10, April.* Bombay: FRCH.

Raphael, D. 2006. "Social determinants of health: present status, unanswered questions, and future directions." *International Journal of Health Services* 36 (4): 651-677.

Razum, O., J. Liyanage, and K. R. Nayar. 2001. "Difficulties in polio eradication." *The Lancet* 357: 476.

Robinson, D. 1980. "The self-help component of primary health care." *Social Science and Medicine* 14 A: 415-421.

Robinson, D. 1981. "Self-help groups in primary health care." *World Health Forum* 2: 185-191.

Rondinelli, D. A. 1983. *Decentralization in developing countries, Staff Working Paper 581.* Washington DC: The World Bank.

Sackett, D. L. W. M. Rosenberg, J. A. Gray, R. B. Haynes, and W. S. Richardson. 1996." Evidence based medicine: What it is and what isn't." *British Medical Journal* 312: 71.

SACOSAN. 2008. *Sustaining the sanitation revolution: India Country Paper.* New Delhi: SACOSAN III.

Saltman, R. B.1995. *Applying planned market logic to developing countries' health system: An initial exploration. Discussion Paper No. 4.* Geneva: World Health Organization, Forum on Health Sector Reform.

Saltman, R. B., V. Bankauskaite, and K. Vrangbaek. 2007. Eds. *Decentralization in health care: strategies and outcomes*. Berkshire: Open University Press.

Saltman, R. B. 2008. "Decentralization, re-centralization and future European health policy." *European Journal of Public Health* 18: 106-108.

Saltman, R. B., A. Duran, and HFW Dubois. 2011. Eds. *Reforming public hospitals: Reform strategies and the movement towards institutional autonomy*. Copenhagen: WHO.

Sarkar, AK. 2005. *NGOs: The new lexicon of health care*. New Delhi: The Concept publishing company.

Satishchandran, T. R. 1993. "Panchayat Raj and health care: the Karnataka experience." In, *People's health in people's hands: a model for Panchayati Raj*, edited by N. H. Antia, and K. Bhatia, 328-35. Bombay: FRCH.

Satishchandran, T. R. 1994. "Inter-tier allocation of functions." In. *Decentralization: Panchayats in the ninties*, edited by A Mukherji, 24-9. New Delhi: Vikas.

Selden, M. 1988. "Household, cooperative, and the state in the remaking of China's countryside." In, *cooperative and collective in China's rural development: between state and private interest,* edited by E. B. Vermeer, F. N. Pieke, and L. W. Chong, 17-45. New York: M.E.Sharp.

Self Employed Women's Association. 2000. *Annual Report –2000*. Ahmedabad: SEWA.

Self Employed Women's Association. 2000. *Promoting health security for women in the informal sector*. Ahemedabad: SEWA.

Self-help Promotion Event Secretariat. 2001. "Development through self-help: be a part of it." ICDDR Social and Behavioral Science Program, Pre-prints of papers of the Self-Help Promotion Conference, Dhaka, 10-11 November 2001.

Sen A. 1999. *Development as freedom*. New Delhi: Oxford University Press.

Sen, B. 2001. "People's health care initiatives in Chattisgarh district, Madhya Pradesh." In, *Public health and the poverty of reforms: the South Asian predicament*, edited by I. Qadeer, K. Sen, and K. R. Nayar, 413-418. New Delhi: Sage.

Sen, K. 2003. "Restructuring health services and policies of privatization- an overview of experience," In *Restructuring health services: changing contexts and comparative perspectives,* edited by K. Sen, 21-32. London: Zed Books.

Sharma, R. 2007. *Sector wise approach in reproductive and child health program in India: a critical review. Unpublished M.Phil dissertation*. New Delhi: Jawaharlal Nehru University.

Shaw, M. 2004. "Housing and public health." *Annual Review of Public Health* 25:397–418.

Shekhar, C., and F. Ram. 2011. *In-depth analysis of equity differences in health outcomes focusing on reproductive and child health in six Indian states, Policy Brief.* Mumbai: IIPS.

Shukla, A., and A. Phadke. 1999. "Health movement in India." *Health Action* 12 (12): 6-9.

Sigamani, P. 2005. *The new public management (NPM): relevance to healthcare services. Unpublished M. Phil dissertation*. New Delhi: Jawaharlal Nehru University.

Sinats, K. 2001. *Health Co-operatives: a viable Solution to the current crisis in Health Service Delivery. British Columbia Institute for Co-operative Studies Occasional Papers 5.* Victoria: British Columbia Institute for Co-operative Studies.

Singer, P. A. A. D. Taylor, A. S. Daar, R. E. Upshur, J. A. Singh, J. V. Lavery. 2007. "Grand Challenges in global health: the ethical, social and cultural program." *PLos Medicine* 4 (9): e265. Accessed 12/12/2007. http://www.plosmedicine.org

Stahl, T., M. Wismar, E. Ollila, E. Lahtinen, and K. Leppo . 2006. *Health in All Policies: Prospects and potentials.* Finland: Ministry of Social Affairs and Health.

Standing, H. 1997. "Gender and equity in health sector reform programs: a review." *Health Policy and Planning* 12: 1-18.

Stefanini, A.1999. "Ethics in health care priority-setting: a north-south double standard?." *Tropical Medicine and International Health* 4: 709-712.

Swaminathan, M. S., and R. V. Bhavani. 2013. "Food production & availability—Essential prerequisites for sustainable food security." *Indian Journal of Medical Research* 138: 383-91.

Swarup, A., and N. Jain. 2012. "Rashtriya Swasthya BimaYojana: A case study from India. Working paper." Accessed 9 March. http://www.rsby.gov.in/Documents.aspx?ID=14

Tandon, R., and R. Mohanty. 2002. *Civil society and governance.* New Delhi: PRIA.

Thankappan, K. R. 2001. "Some health implications of globalisation in Kerala, India." *Bulletin of the World Health Organisation* 79: 892-93.

Travis, P., S. Bennett, A. Haynes, T. Pang, Z. Bhutta, A. A. Hyder, N. R. Pielemeier, A. Mills, and T. Evans. 2004. "Overcoming health-systems constraints to achieve the Millennium Development Goals." *The Lancet* 364: 901-906.

UNRISD. 2000. *Visible hands: taking responsibility for social development.* Geneva: Geneva 2000 Forum.

UNFPA. 2009. *Concurrent assessment of JSY in selected states.* New Delhi: UNFPA.

UNICEF. 2009. *Coverage evaluation survey report 2009.* New Delhi: UNICEF and Government of India.

United Nations. 1997. *Cooperative enterprise in the health and social care sectors. A Global Survey.* New York: UN Department for Policy Coordination and Sustainable Development

United Nations. 2001. *Cooperatives in social development: report of the Secretary-General.* Geneva: ECOSOC.

Update. 2005. "India's huge market for low-cost health insurance." *Micro health insurance update* 2: 1.

Victor, R. G. 1962. "Report on medical care programs in India." In, *Report of the Health Survey and Planning Committee, Vol.2, Appendices*, edited by Government of India, 35-64. New Delhi: Ministry of Health and Family Welfare.

Walker D., C. Champion, S. Hossain, T. Wahed, R. Gazi, T. P. Koehlmoos, D. Asiimwe, M. K. Ranson, and S. Bennett. 2009. *Establishing non-state sector research priorities in developing countries using a participatory methodology.* Geneva: Alliance for Health Policy and Systems Research and WHO.

Walt G., J. Shiffman, H. Schneider, S. F. Murray, R. Brugha, and L. Gilson. 2008. "'Doing' health policy analysis: methodological and conceptual reflections and challenges." *Health Policy and Planning* 23: 308-317.

WHO. 1978. *Primary Health care, report of the International Conference on Primary Health Care, Alma-Ata, 6-12 September, 1978.* Geneva: WHO

WHO. 1986. *Ottawa Charter for health promotion.* Copenhagen: WHO

WHO. 2007. *World Health Statistics.* Geneva: WHO

WHO and PHAC- Public Health Agency of Canada. 2008. *Health equity through intersectoral action: an analysis of 18 country casestudies.* Geneva: WHO

WHO and PHAC- Public Health Agency of Canada. 2008. *Health equity through intersectoral action: an analysis of 18 country case studies.* Geneva: WHO.

WHO. 2008. *Commission social determinants of health. Closing the gap in a generation: Health equity through action on the social determinants of health.* Geneva: WHO.

WHO. 2010. *Adelaide statement on health in all policies.* Adelaide: WHO and Government of South Australia.

WHO-Government of India Biennial work plan. 2012. *The role of intersectoral action in implementing the Framework Convention for Tobacco Control in India. Final draft version* (made available through WHO SEARO).

Wilkinson, R. G. 1996. *Unhealthy societies. The afflictions of inequality.* London: Routledge.

Wolfe, M. 1994. *Social integration: institutions and actors. Occasional Paper No.4. World Summit for Social Development.* Geneva: United Nations Research Institute for Social Development.

World Bank. 1993. *Investing in health. World Development Report 1993.* New York: Oxford University Press.

World Bank. 2006. *Equity and Development. World Development Report 2006.* New York: Oxford University Press.

World Bank. 2013. Accessed 29 Aug http://www1.worldbank.org/publicsector/decentralization/what.htm

WSP., and Government of India. 2011. *Towards drinking water security in India: lessons from the field.* New Delhi: Water and Sanitation Program, The World Bank and Ministry of Rural Development.

Xiao-ming, C., T. Hu, and Z. Lin. 1993. "The rise and decline of the cooperative medical system in rural China." *International Journal of Health Services* 23: 731-742.

Xing-Yuan G., and T. Sheng-Lan. 1995. Reforms of the Chinese health care financing system. *Health Policy* 32: 181-91.

Yunguo, L., and G. Bloom. 2002. *Designing a rural health reform project: the negotiation of change in China. IDS Working Paper 150.* Sussex: Institute of Development Studies.

Zhu, NS., Z. H. Ling, J. Shen, J. M. Lane, and S. L. Hu. 1989. "Factors associated with the decline of the cooperative medical system and barefoot doctors in rural China." *Bulletin of World Health Organization* 67: 431-41.

Index

Alliance for Health Policy and Systems Research, 82, 83, 115, 136
Anglemyer, A., 62
Araujo, J J.r, 84
Archard, L., 124
Arhin-Tenkorang, D., 58
Asian Development Bank, 45, 46
Asiatic mode of market orientation, 9–10
Aslimwe, D., 136
Athreya, VB., 131
Attanayake, N., 85
Attwood DW., 121
Aziz, A., 86

Baker, PI., 34
Bali, N., 122
Bambra, C., 66
Bandopaddhyay, D., 88
Banerji, D., 1, 25, 44, 74, 141,142
Bankauskaite, V., 82
Bao-Gang, S., 120
Bardhan, P., 84, 94
Basu, SK., 74
Baviskar, BS., 121
Beaglehole, R., 52, 70
behavior; change communication, 29, 67–68; happiness, 67; individual orientation, 69, 71, 72, 132, 135; psyche, 70
Bell, J., 52
Bennett, S., 54, 136
Bernstein, A., 52
Bero, L., 62
Beteille, A., 114
Bhatt, ER., 122
Bhatt, R., 24
Bhattacharya, S., 4
Bhavani, RV., 35
Bhore committee, 10–11, 12, 20, 24, 36, 37, 41, 48–49, 58, 111, 140–141
Bhuiya, A., 129
Bhutta, Z., 54
Birn, Anne-Emanuelle., 52
Blomstedt, Y., 70
Bloom, G., 84, 119, 120
Boerma, T., 144
Bogg, L., 120
Bonita, R., 70
Borysiewicz, LK., 52
Bossert, T., 82
Bowen, S., 67
Brenieman, L., 126
Brugha, R., 5
Byass, P 70

Cai, W. 120
Cao, H., 119
Cardosi, J., 39
Carr-Hill, R., 47
Carrin, G., 58, 119, 120
Cassels, A., 47, 48
Chambers, R., 40
Champion, C., 136
Chadha committee, 13, 14
Chase, E., 47
Chowdhury, R., 129
Chuengsatiansup, K., 113
civil society, 2, 5, 6, 7, 78, 86, 98, 107, 116, 127, 136, 141, 144, 146; NGO and health, 113–117
Coffey, D., 35
Colagiuri, S., 52
Collins, C., 84
communicable diseases, 13, 16, 32, 35, 46, 49, 50, 52, 91, 94, 99, 143
Coombes, Y., 39
co-operatives, 25, 110, 113, 117–118, 128, 129, 130; in developing countries, 118–120; in Gujrat and Kerala, 120–121; health co-operatives, 121–122; SEWA, 122; Medical co-operatives, 122–125
cost-effectiveness, 17, 31, 41, 54, 81, 115, 125, 129, 132, 135
Coutinho, L., 113
CSDH, 104, 144

Daar, AS., 52, 53
Das, A., 29
Das, J., 62
Das, MK., 94
Das, RK., 113
Das, V., 113
Dasgupta, R., 26
de-centralization; approaches, 82–83; market-driven, 83; international experience, 84;Indian case, 85–87; conceptual issues, 87; people's planning, 90–94; community innovation, 96–100; methodology, 100–103; focused action and collective mobilization, 103–107
Devine, J., 39
disorder, definition, 140; categories, 140–143; new documentation, 144; disorder to stability, 145
Djurfeldt, G., 4, 74, 131
Doherty, J., 5
Dong, H 120
Drasser, K., 62
Dreze, J., 85
Dror, D., 58
Dubois, HFW., 95
Dubos, R., 71
Dubowitz, T., 34
Duran, A., 95

ECCP project, 59, 60
Edwards, M., 113
epidemiological, 2, 9, 19, 24, 30, 32, 39, 41, 51, 52, 55, 69, 74, 91, 92, 96, 105, 107, 140, 144
Estes, CL., 84
European Union., 100
Evans, DB., 144
Evans, T., 54
evidence-based medicine, 66; eminence based, 41, 66

Feng, X., 119
Finegood, DT., 52
Fishbein, M., 68
Franco, TD., 128, 129
Friberg, P., 70
Friel, S., 34
Fu, W., 120

Gilson, L., 5
Glass, RI., 52
Global HIV prevention working group, 68
Gopalan, C., 35
Gakidou, E., 28
Ganguly, N., 2
Gautam, M., 11

Gazi, R., 136
gender, 2, 26, 32, 51, 57, 69, 70, 73, 74, 91, 99, 100, 102, 128, 129, 131
George, J., 91
George, MV., 123
George, S., 121
Gerein, N., 82
goal-setting in health, 48–53
Government of Chattisgarh, 100
Government of Gujarat, 100
Government of India, 10, 11,12, 13, 14, 15, 18, 19, 20, 21, 23, 25, 27, 27, 28, 30,31 ,32, 36, 39, 40, 49, 50, 51, 52, 59, 63, 64, 77, 79, 87, 95, 100, 111, 112, 115, 116, 117, 121, 130, 140
Government of Kerala, 60, 90, 104, 123, 124, 131
Government of Madhya Pradesh, 99
Government of Odisha, 98
Government of Uttar Pradesh, 68
Gray, JA., 66
Green, A., 82, 84, 114, 115
Grossman, A., 39
Gu, Y., 119
Gupta, A., 35
Gupta, D., 134

Hagopian, A., 29
Haines, A., 26
Hanson, K., 124
Hao, Y., 120
Haynes, A., 54
Haynes, RB., 66
health for all, 16, 49–50, 141
health in all, 39, 75, 77, 80; Adelaide statement, 78
health insurance,10, 11, 12, 13, 15, 20, 21, 22, 23, 24, 25, 29, 40, 48, 58–62, 65, 78, 97, 118, 120, 121, 125, 126; RSBY, 24, 61–62, 97
health policy analysis, 5
health promotion, 32, 33, 128; Ottawa charter, 71
health reforms, milestones, 44–45; doctrine, 45–47; enzymatic, 6; cocktail, 9, 15, 29, 41, 143. *see also*, structural adjustment
health services development, vii, 1, 9, 10, 26, 31, 43, 44, 51, 86; actors, 5
health system, 1, 2, 4, 5, 6, 18, 27, 30, 50, 54, 79, 82, 83, 90, 98, 115, 127, 136
Heller, PS., 58
Helliwell, J., 67
Hertzman, C., 74
HIV/AIDS, 20, 53, 61, 68, 143
Hobsbawm, EJ., 140, 141
Hogan, MC., 8
Hoisington, JA., 28
Holst, J., 46
homogenization of order, 139
Hong, W., 119, 120
Horvath, T., 62
Hossain, S., 136
housing, 1, 35, 36–37, 41, 75, 76, 77, 78, 87, 111
Hsiao, WC., 58, 59, 120
Hsu, J., 144
Hu, S., 120
Hu, SL., 119
Hu, T., 119, 120
Hui, Y., 119, 120
Hunter, DJ., 2,5,143
Huss, R., 82
Hussi, P., 126
Hutchinson, L. 104
Hyden, G., 121
Hyder, AA., 54

ICSSR-ICMR committee, 16–17, 41, 141
India vision, 21
Indian public health standard, 32, 63–64
Indian theory of communication, 69
institutional delivery, 20, 26, 27, 28, 63, 69, 99; Kerala, 96; Jharkhand, 98; Odisha, 98; Chattisgarh, 100

integrated approach, 13, 14, 33, 36, 39, 54, 65, 69, 77
interdisciplinary framework, 2–3, 5
International Co-operative Information Centre., 117
International Institute for Population Sciences., 55, 56, 57
intersectoral, 34, 70; approach, 75–79
Irwin, LG., 74

Jacob, S., 34
Jaffri, A., 88, 89
Jain, N., 61
Jakab, M., 58
James, KS., 102
James, SL., 28
janani suraksha yojana (JSY), 26, 27, 98, 99; performance, 27–29
Jayaseelan, J., 127
Jeffrey, P., 26
Jeffrey, R., 26
Jhabvala, R., 122
Jiaying, C., 119, 120
Jobert, B.,45
Jun, Y., 119, 120
Jungalwalla committee, 14, 150

Kalpana, K., 128, 129
Karmakar, KG., 128
Karpagam, S., 82
Kartar Singh committee, 14–15
Katz, AH., 127
Kaviraj, S., 109
Kawanga, M., 83
Kennedy, GE., 62
Khilnani, S., 110
Kilby, P., 114
Kinlaw, HS., 62
Koehlmoos, TP., 136
Koplan, J., 52
Kothari, R., 85
Krieger, N., 4, 71
Krishnamurty, HR., 29
KSSP, 60, 80, 135
Kullmann, C., 39
Kumar, CA., 39
Kutzin, J., 144
Kyobutungi, C., 127, 129, 131, 132, 134

LaFond, AK., 104
Lagarde, M., 26
Lahtinen, E., 77
Lalit, D., 28
Lane, JM., 119
Lavery, JV., 53
Layard, R., 67
Leino, J., 62
Leppo, K., 77
Levinson, D., 34
Lewis, D., 113
Licheng, Z., 119, 120
Lim, SS., 28
Lin, Z., 119, 120
Lindberg, O., 126
Lindberg, S., 4, 74, 131
Ling, ZH 119
Linkins, KW., 84
Liu, X., 119
Liu, XZ., 119
Liu, Y., 120
Liyanage, J., 25
Lucas, H, 120
Luiz, AC., 84

macro economics and health, national commission, 21–22
Mahipal., 94
managerial phase, 24–26
Marmot, M., 71
Mathew, G., 85
Mathur, K., 87, 104
Matthews, DR., 52
Matthias, A., 114, 115
Mayoux, L., 128
McIntyre, D., 144
McKeown, T., 71
McPake, B., 124
Medeazza, GV., 40
Messenger, S., 4
Michaud, C., 115

millennium development goals, 28, 70, 72, 96, 105, 143; emergence of, 53–54; *see also*, goal-setting in health
Mills, A., 54, 144
Mishra, US., 102
Mladovsky, P., 59
modernizing government program, 46–47; *see also,* new public management
Mohanty, R., 110
Montagu, DD., 62
Moore, M., 43, 45, 47
Mossialos, E., 59
Mudaliar committee, 12–13
Mukerji committee, 13–14
Mukherjee, N., 39, 88
Mukhopadhyay, A., 32, 33
Murphy, J., 126
Murray, CJL., 115
Murray, SF., 5
Mushtaque, A., 129
Mykhalovskiy, E., 3

Nabel, EG., 52
Naidoo, K., 110
Nair, S., 54
Nambiar, ACK., 124
Narayana, D., 61
national planning committee, 12, 36, 111
national health policy, 17, 18, 23, 24
national rural health mission, 9–10, 11, 21, 22, 25, *41*, 45, 68, 69, 82, 94, 95, 96, 103, 143
Navarro, V., 3,4
Nayar, KR., 2, 17, 25, 26, 36, 37, 41, 48, 54, 64, 72, 77, 87, 88, 91, 96, 105, 113, 117, 122, 123, 125, 126, 127, 129, 131, 132, 134, 141
Nayar, PKB., 109
neo-liberalism, 22, 26, 29, 40, 54, 87, 89, 103, 114, 134, 136, 137, 139, 145, 146; new forms, 58, 62, 67,
new public health, 1
new public management, 46–47, 94–95, 143
ninth plan, 18, 20, 23, 38, 39
non-communicable diseases, 20, 29–32, 35, 50, 52, 53, 65, 70, 143
non-state sector, 136, 137
nutrition, 1, 16, 17, 33, 34–35, 40, 50, 53, 63, 68, 69, 72, 96, 97, 99, 113, 131; ICDS, 34, 97; mid-day meal, 34, 77

Ollila, E., 77
Osborne, K., 127
outline, of the book, 5; theoretical position, 5–6; methodology, 5
Overy C., 4

Palacios, R., 61
Palmer, N., 26
Pang, T., 54
Panikkar, PGK., 91, 123
Patnaik, U., 145, 146
people's movement, 135–136
Perez, E., 39
Persad, DL., 52
Peterman, JN., 34
Phadke, A., 135, 136
PHFI, 78, 144
PHM, 143
Pielemeier, NR., 54
Pieterse, JN., 142
planning commission, evaluation study, 18 19
political economy framework, 3–5, 43
Prakash, M., 39
Pramming, SK., 52
Prasad, NP., 62
Preker, AS., 58
primary health care, 3, 17, 18, 32, 41, 44, 48, 49, 53, 65, 77, 80, 85, 92, 94, 105, 112, 122, 127, 130, 132, 133, 141
public-private partnership, 6, 45, 46, 61, 62–63, 65, 89, 114, 125, 144
Purdom, W., 36
Purohit, BC., 124

Qadeer, I., 1, 2, 17, 26, 48, 64, 65, 113
Qicheng, J., 119, 120

Raghavendra, P., 62
Rajagopal., 128
Rajagopal, A., 131
Ram, F., 28
Ramachandran, P., 35
Ramani, K., 82
Ranson, MK., 136
Rao, D., 29
Rao, S., 88
Raphael, D., 72
Razum, O., 25, 72, 117, 125, 126, 127, 129, 132
reproductive and child health, 160; program, 50–53
Richardson, WS., 66
Ritu Priya., 2
Robiarto, A., 39
Robinson, D., 127
Ron, A., 119, 120
Rondinelli, DA., 82
Rosenberg, WM., 66
Rutherford, GW., 62

Sachs, J 67
Sackett, DL., 66
SACOSAN., 40
Saltman, RB., 45, 81, 82, 95
sanitation, 1, 11, 16, 33, 35, 36, 37, 38, 41, 49, 53, 63, 68, 87, 91, 95, 98, 99, 111, 113; program, 39–40; total sanitation, 78; sanitation committee, 39, 95
Sarkar, AK., 113
Sarna, G., 52
Sarrafzadegan, N; 52
Satishchandran, TR., 87, 88
Schneider, H., 5
Schultink, W., 34
Segall, M., 119
Selden, M., 117, 119
Self Employed Women's Association (SEWA), 122, 125, 128, 129, 132
self-help, 7, 10, 15, 16, 36, 41, 47, 97, 111, 117,122, 125, 126–127; in South Asia, 127–129; under NGO sponsorship, 129–130; under government sponsorship,130–131; typology, 132, 133; facilitating factors, 135
Self-help Promotion Event Secretariat, 129, 130
Sen, A., 74, 85
Sen, B., 103
Sen, K., 48, 55, 113
Setiawan, D., 39
Shah, N., 62
Sharma, R., 50
Shaw, M., 37
Shekhar, C., 28
Shen, J., 119
Sheng-Lan, T., 119
Shi, L., 4
Shiffman, J., 5
Shrivastav committee, 15–16, 17, 18
Shukla, A., 135, 136
Shuo, Z., 119, 120
Shyamprasad, KM., 11
Siddiqi, A., 74
Sigamani, P., 46, 95
Sinats, K., 117
Singer, PA., 52, 53
Singh, JA., 53
Singh, U., 39
Smith, R., 52
social determinants, 2, 3, 4, 49, 54, 80, 106, 144; approach, 71–73; embodiment, 4, 105, 155; *see also* social disparities
social disparities, 54; caste, 2, 26, 27–28, 36, 55–58, 89, 91, 99, 102; social exclusion, 55, 71, 74, 107
social science, 2, 4, 49, 95
Sokhey committee, 12, 111
Soman, CR., 91, 123
Stahl, T., 77
Standing, H., 84
Stefanini, A., 134

Stordalen, G., 70
structural adjustment, 4, 24, 26, 47–48, 81, 87, 89, 93, 113, 128, 139
Sudarshan, H., 82
Swaminathan, MS., 35
Swarup, A., 61

Tandon, R., 110
Tang, S., 119
Taylor, AD., 53
techno-centric, 1, 40, 49, 52, 65
teleology, 6, 7, 146
tenth plan, 23, 39
the tobacco control, 29, 78–79
third sector organization, 136, 137
Thankappan, KR., 124
Tiwari, M., 62
Tomson, G., 82
Travis, P., 54
Tuohong, Z., 119, 120
twelfth plan, 29, 30, 32, 39

UNFPA., 27, 99
UNICEF., 27, 49, 50
United Nations., 53, 72, 117, 118, 121
UNRISD., 115
universal health care, 83, 141, 144, 145
Update., 60
Upshur, RE., 53

Verma, G., 34
Victor, RG., 121
Vidyasagar, R., 131
Vonod, D., 120
Vrangbaek, K., 82

Wahed, T., 136
Walker, D., 136
Wall, S., 70
Walt, G., 5
Wang, JL., 119
Wang, K., 120
Wartono, D., 39
water supply, 37–39, 41, 50, 75
Weir, L., 3
WHO, 49, 72, 73, 74, 77, 144
WHO and PHAC, 75, 107
WHO-Government of India biennial work plan, 79
Wilkinson, RG., 71
Wismar, M., 77
Wolfe, M., 115
World Bank, 13, 23, 24, 39, 40, 45, 48, 58, 59, 73, 81, 82, 83, 87, 143
WSP and Government of India, 39

Xiao-ming, C., 119, 120
Xing-Yuan, G., 84, 119, 120
Xuesheng, L., 119, 120

Yach, D., 52
Yide, Y., 119, 120
Yunguo, L., 120

Zhaoyang, Z., 119, 120
Zhu, NS., 119
Zwi, AB., 67

About the Author

Kesavan Rajasekharan Nayar is chief fellow at Santhigiri Social Research Institute. He taught public health at Jawaharlal Nehru University for twenty-eight years and has been DAAD guest professor at Heidelberg University. He is the author of *Ecology and Health: A Systems Approach* and coeditor of *Public Health and the Poverty of Reforms: The South Asian Predicament.*

www.ingramcontent.com/pod-product-compliance
Lightning Source LLC
Chambersburg PA
CBHW051251200926
51612CB00001B/10